There's No Place Like Home...
for Sex Education

Dedication

This book is dedicated to all young people who deserve honest, affirming sex education, and to parents who are doing their very best to support and love them.

There's No Place Like Home... for Sex Education

A guidebook for parents

by Mary Gossart

Spanish edition available

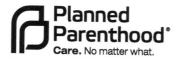

Planned Parenthood®
Care. No matter what.

Planned Parenthood of Southwestern Oregon

Published by Planned Parenthood of Southwestern Oregon

Planned Parenthood of Southwestern Oregon
3579 Franklin Blvd., Eugene OR 97403
www.ppsworegon.org

Illustrations by Regina Gelfer, Gelfer Graphics
Cover and interior design by Monserrat Garcia
Book production by Joanna Bartlett, Alight Communication
Printed in the United States of America

First edition, 1988
Second edition, 2002
Third edition, February 2015

Library of Congress Control Number: 2015932119

ISBN 978-0-578-15744-3

Contents

Contents

Introduction

Parents matter. The conversations they have with their children matter. *There's No Place Like Home... for Sex Education* is a practical guide that helps parents talk with their children about sexual issues in open, thoughtful, effective ways.

Studies show that parent-child connectedness and good communication about sexuality has positive effects for young people. It helps them form their personal values, make good sexual decisions and protect their own sexual health. While there are many possible sources of sexual information (and *mis*information!) – including school, peers, faith leaders, media, the Internet and more – national surveys are clear: Teens want their parents to talk with them about these issues, and they want their parents' guidance.

Parents have a unique and important role in educating their children about sex. In fact, teens say that their parents have the greatest influence on their decisions about relationships, love and sex. Yet many moms and dads (as well as grandparents, guardians and others who may be parenting children) find themselves challenged and unprepared to have these conversations. They may not feel confident about their own information. They may assume that their children are too young and not realize that sex education begins at birth. Some worry that talking about sex somehow encourages young people to experiment, or that it puts ideas into their heads that they otherwise would not have. Parents may not have a model in their own lives for what it looks like, sounds like and feels like to have positive, appropriate discussions with their children about sexuality.

There's No Place Like Home... for Sex Education offers a model and is centered around the understanding that:

- Sexual learning is a life-long process. Children are absorbing sexual messages, attitudes and values from the moment they are born.

- Children need and deserve information about sexuality throughout their growing up years. It makes great sense to give thoughtful attention to how that happens.

- Parents are an important and influential part of their children's sex education.

Using this book

There's No Place Like Home... for Sex Education contains individual sections that are organized by age/grade levels. The book can be read from start to finish, or you can skip around to various ages and topics that are relevant for your family at this time.

Each section looks at questions, behaviors and issues related to sexuality that are typical for young people or important to address with them during that developmental stage. There are also sample conversations throughout. These are simply intended to provide ideas for content and language that you can use for a variety of questions, topics and settings. Of course, every young person is unique. As a parent, you are in the best position to know how to introduce these conversations within your own family.

Effective parent-child communication about sexuality is not about making our way through a laundry list and checking off each item once we have talked about it. Conversations about the very same topic happen more than once. As with all important learning, the lessons and discussions are ongoing and reinforced throughout our children's growing up years. Specific issues that were introduced when our children were younger become more immediate or relevant as they develop physically, intellectually, emotionally and socially. Because of that, you will notice that a number of themes and topics are revisited throughout several sections of the book. This is intentional. The design also helps fulfill one of the book's objectives, which is that any age/grade section can be read on its own and make sense without having to read through the previous pages.

A word about pronouns: You will also notice a variety of pronouns used when referring to young people in this book rather than defaulting to a single gender (such as "he," "his" and "him") or the awkward "he or she," "his or her," "her or him." Occasionally you will see "s/he" as shorthand for "he or she." At times in this book, the pronouns "they," "their" and "them" are used in reference to a single individual. This is intended to be more inclusive and to respectfully acknowledge that not all people identify with the male or female gender classification. Rather, there is a spectrum of gender identities.

A word about words: The language used in sexuality education is often interpreted in different ways by different people. Rather than leave understanding to chance, here are a few definitions of language and concepts as used in this book:

- **Biological sex** – the gender a person is assigned at birth (this is usually done visually… and sometimes the assignment turns out to be incorrect); beyond sexual anatomy, biological sex is determined by a person's chromosomes and hormones.

- **Body image** – how someone feels about their body; the level of personal comfort and satisfaction they have with how their body looks and feels.

- **Gender binary** – a social system that classifies people as either distinctly male or distinctly female.

- **Gender expression** – the ways a person conveys their sense of their gender to others (for example – how they dress, look, act, etc.).

- **Gender identity** – a person's inner sense of being male, female, somewhere in between, or outside of the gender binary. This may be the same as or different than the gender they were assigned at birth.

- **Gender nonconforming** – by nature or by choice, not following others' expectations or stereotypes of how someone should act based on the gender they were assigned at birth (sometimes referred to as **gender variant or diverse**).

- **Sex (as in "having sex")** – people define having sex in different ways. Examples include vaginal intercourse, anal intercourse, mouth to genitals or anus, and genital-to-genital rubbing.

- **Sexual orientation** – refers to the gender or genders to which a person is physically and romantically attracted.

- **Sexual protection** – barrier methods such as condoms and dental dams that are used when having sex to help prevent the transmission of sexually transmitted diseases.

- **Sexuality** – dimension of human beings that includes many parts such as body awareness, relationships, intimacy, sexual identity, sexual health and reproduction.

- **Sexuality education** – teachings that address the many aspects of human sexuality (sometimes referred to as **sex education**).

Littles and **Preschoolers**

Sex education??? My child's only 3 years old!

Well then, already s/he has received a wealth of messages about sexuality – at least three years worth, in fact. Just think about it:

- When infants are touched and cuddled, they learn about love… and that they are loved. Nurturing touch, connection, bonding and loving relationships – yes! – these are all parts of sexuality education for little ones, and perhaps the most fundamental pieces.

- Choices of clothing, colors, toys and playtime activities send early messages about gender assumptions, roles and expectations. Are you expanding your children's choices and exposure beyond what's considered conventional or acceptable for each gender? Or are you narrowing the options – even unintentionally?

- Seeing a brother, sister or parent in the shower teaches children about physical differences among people.

- Bathing, diapering and potty training are perfect opportunities to name body parts. Have you been as enthusiastic about naming your little one's penis or vulva as you have about the fingers and toes (which affirms that *all* of our body parts are special and important to know about)? Or do you tend to skip over that section of the body or simply bundle the genitals into a vague term like "your private parts" (which your child might take to mean that somehow these body parts are not OK... or not OK to talk about)?

- When you show a willingness to simply and honestly answer questions like, *"How did the baby get in the mommy?"* it provides a lot more than just information. It also conveys a feeling about the subject of sex. It sends the message, *"That's an important question and I want to talk with you about it."*

You have been educating your child about sexuality all along, through your words as well as your silence, in your verbal and nonverbal communication.

You have been educating your child about sexuality all along, through your words as well as your silence, in your verbal and nonverbal communication. Your responses and reactions have taught your child a great deal about sexuality – not only in terms of information, but also in terms of your comfort, values and attitudes.

You cannot avoid being your child's primary and most important sex educator... nor would you want to. You're an important influence as your child develops sexual understanding and attitudes. The family experiences you shape, from the moment your child is born, help determine the extent to which s/he develops positive, healthy feelings about sexuality. Yet the thought that sex education begins at birth is a novel idea to many parents. It's just not something we tend to think about when our children are newborns or infants.

The unsuspecting parent may find that several formative years have passed before the realization sets in: **even very young children deserve thoughtful, intentional sexuality education**. Children do better when we talk early and often with them, listen to them, share information coupled with personal values, and create an environment in which talking about sexual issues is normal, comfortable and expected.

When my child asks, then we'll talk

But will you recognize the asking? Children wonder about lots of things – including sexuality – long before they can verbalize the questions. For example, a little one may want to watch daddy in the shower or touch mommy's pregnant belly. These are ideal "teachable moments" to pass along brief lessons on anatomy, reproduction and birth. They also give you a chance to reaffirm that sexually is an appropriate topic to discuss within the family. All these things help build an atmosphere of comfort and trust that encourages children to turn to their parents when they have questions now and in the future.

Concerned about telling your child too much too soon? S/he will simply take in what s/he can, and let you know when the conversation's over or getting too long or complex (watch for glassy eyes, yawning, changing the subject, leaving the scene, etc.). S/he may not have been interested in all the detail, but your comments aren't wasted. You've let your child know that you're there, you're approachable and you're happy to talk about this important topic.

So what about gender roles?

By the age of 2, many children have formed a pretty good idea about what it means to be a boy or a girl… or at least what the culture expects that being a boy or girl is all about. Throughout this time, the people in their lives and the environment around them have been providing cues about what it means to be male or female… and what are considered suitable behaviors for their gender. Let's be cautious about putting our children into one of two boxes.

When we avoid pigeonholing male/female behaviors, expectations and roles, children learn that their life experiences and options need not be limited by gender. Take advantage of the many simple opportunities to broaden your child's perspective and accept them for who they are:

- **Share** household chores.

- **Encourage** children to play with toys and take part in games or activities that cross traditional gender lines. (Check out this YouTube clip of a little girl who has some pretty strong views about gender stereotyping: https://www.youtube.com/watch?v=-CU04OHqbas)

- **Read** stories that feature people with different genders in a variety of roles.

- **Pay attention to language** that opens up options for all genders (such as "firefighter" rather than "fireman"). Use a variety of pronouns ("he," "she," "they") when talking about leaders, dancers, scientists, caregivers, etc.

- **Allow your child to express the gender that feels right to them.**

There is a great range of interests and behaviors for all genders. It's also important to appreciate that for some, gender identity doesn't fit neatly into the gender binary (you're either male or female). We're learning to think more about gender as falling on a spectrum, and respecting that some of our children experience a blending of gender characteristics. And some children are born with bodies whose internal and/ or external organs or sex chromosomes convey a mix of features labeled as male or female. We're becoming more aware of the astounding complexities of gender and the grand diversity among humans.

Amidst all this, one thing is both simple and true: Our children flourish when we allow them to be who they are, and when we love, accept and embrace them for it.

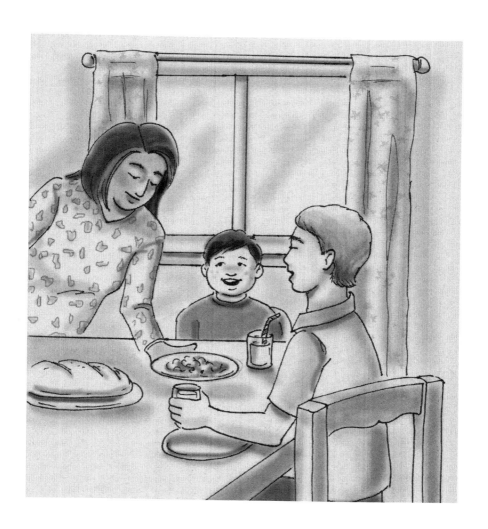

An ear is an ear...

...And a penis is a penis, not a "wee-wee;" a vulva is a vulva, not a "down there." The popular generic phrase "private parts" may feel more comfortable to a parent, but it's incomplete... and let's be honest: it's a way to avoid saying the *real* words. Using vague language or inventing terms for sexual body parts can send the message that they're somehow different, or that there's something wrong or unmentionable about them. That's one way children learn to be embarrassed and awkward about their genitals. If your child refers to sexual body parts using slang s/he's heard from friends, consider saying something like, *"Some people may call it that... the real name is penis."* It's a simple, matter-of-fact, no big deal response that packs an important message.

Studies have shown the value of teaching children accurate names for sexual body parts. It normalizes the use of those terms and promotes respect and a positive attitude about bodies and sexuality. And then there are those painfully difficult times when the understanding and use of accurate terms is especially critical. If a child is trying to describe an injury or inappropriate sexual touch, s/he needs to be equipped with language more precise than "down there."

What's that???

Most young children are intensely curious about bodies — and not just their own. There's particular fascination with gender differences and body functions. Their interest pops up in a variety of ways: "playing doctor," wanting to watch mom or dad in the bathroom, genital play, comparing body parts to friends or siblings of another gender.

A little girl might wonder what happened to her penis, or a boy might point to mommy's breasts and ask, *"What are those?"* Opportunities abound for sharing information about sexuality, growth and development.

Q. What happened to my penis?

A. Some people are born with bodies that have a penis. Some people are born with bodies that have another part called a clitoris. You have a clitoris.

Q. How does the baby come out?

A. There are different ways that can happen. Sometimes the baby comes out through an opening called the vagina. Would you like to look at a book about how some babies are born?

Q. Why does Henry stand up to pee and I have to sit?

A. Different bodies are made to urinate – or pee – in different ways. Henry urinates from his penis. You have a small opening in your body near the vagina. You urinate through that opening.

Q. Can I have a baby when I get big?

A. You can certainly be a daddy when you grow up if you want to, Gabe.

Those are just some ideas for simple answers to typical questions that come up at this age. You will decide for yourself how you wish to have these conversations. The important thing is to respond in a supportive way, and not wonder or fret about whether your child understands it all. You're building foundations and creating an environment of open communication within your family. It's a nice time to get a little practice. Take advantage of the easy questions now... it will help you prepare for the more complex ones later on.

Storks and cabbage patches

A little one's view of the world is quite literal. Here's an example: If a baby grows in someone's "tummy," what happens when that person eats lunch? Does the food get all mushed up with the baby in the same place? Confusing, right? One of the benefits of simple, *accurate* answers is that they help avoid confusion.

What about the child who has been told by her parent that the stork delivers babies… and then she later discovers what really happens? How might that color the expectation of trust and honesty between the child and parent? Through our words and behaviors, let the message be: In our family, sex is something we talk about in an open, truthful way.

Children deserve honest answers to their questions — scaled to an appropriate level of understanding, of course. If a young child asks, *"Where did I come from?"* a parent might say, *"What a good question! Do you have any ideas about that?"* This accomplishes a few things: it applauds the child for asking; it can clarify what the question really is (s/he might simply be wondering *where* s/he was born); it buys a bit of time for the parent to gather his thoughts; and it may offer some hints about how much the child already knows. So it helps establish a starting place for giving the most relevant answer.

One response could be something simple and honest: *"You started as a tiny cell. You grew and grew until you were ready to be born."* This alone may satisfy (or not), yet it leaves the door open for more questions and lets the child guide the direction of the conversation. As s/he asks more questions, you can share more details. That information is tailored to a family's specific situation with a continuous eye toward being honest, accurate, straightforward and encouraging. For example, in one family, it may be appropriate to substitute, *"…you grew inside mommy's body in a special place called the uterus."* Not all families are created in that way. So it's important to tell a child what is true for him and his beginning.

The point is that honesty really is the best policy. At this stage there's certainly no need to deliver a lengthy description of intercourse, conception and birth... or, depending on your family's experience, sperm donors, alternative insemination, or surrogate or birth parents. That's not what your little one is interested in now. S/he's just looking for some basic information.

So relax. For a young child, sex doesn't have the same big, emotional significance it does for adults. It's helpful to keep that in mind as you encounter the typical sexual curiosities that come up for your children.

There's a time and place... or is there?

Young children touch their genitals for many reasons. It may be that it comforts them when they are feeling sleepy or bored, nervous or upset. It can happen while they are listening to a story in circle time or absorbed in a television show. Even at this age, it feels good. A parent might find it hard to acknowledge that children are sexual beings or that genital touch and masturbation are a normal part of development. But most experts agree that this can be a healthy expression of sexuality, regardless of age.

The way parents react to their child's genital play is important. Punishing, scolding or pulling the child's hand away with no explanation suggests that this behavior is bad or dirty. A parent's angry reaction can result in their child feeling ashamed and embarrassed. Simply telling the child, *"STOP THAT!"* or trying to distract them with another activity won't be useful for them either.

Most parents do not object to their children's genital play... and yet they want to discourage it, say, in the middle of the grocery store. How does this sound? *"Hayden, I know it feels good when you touch your (penis/clitoris/fill in the blank). Please don't do that now. It's something you do in private — not where other people can see you."* This sends a message about appropriate behavior in public and respect for others. At the same time, it keeps sexuality in a positive light.

Some parents worry that their child is "doing it too much." Children will stop when they are satisfied or if they become physically uncomfortable. On the other hand, compulsive masturbation – or compulsive anything – may signal a problem. If a parent notices his child is masturbating to the point where it interferes with other normal activities, it's time to consult a physician or other professional.

Sexuality is no secret to a 4-year-old

Parents begin teaching their children about sexuality from the moment they are born. Showing love and affection to children – touching, hugging, cuddling – are all ways of giving positive messages about sexuality. How parents respond (or don't respond) to a child's natural curiosity about things like gender differences, body parts and where babies come from certainly implies some pretty clear messages about sexuality.

Children get plenty of sex "education" beyond the home front as well – some of it pretty awful, or at least questionable. There's a daily barrage of media messages about sexuality from billboards, TV, the Internet, magazines and music.

You may think your 4-year-old is oblivious to these messages. S/he isn't. So why not use these as opportunities to talk with your child, provide information, and share your own thoughts and values? At this age your child may not fully understand your message, but one thing will be clear: Mom and/or dad think it's important to talk openly and honestly about these issues.

Even at preschool, children share lots of *mis*information about sex with each other. Some of their ideas can be wild... and they may not check them out with you. So considering all this sex education that goes on with or without a parent being aware of it, you want to get your 2 cents in too!

Show me yours... I'll show you mine

Hmmm. Carolina and her little friend Will are playing quietly in the other room — a little too quietly. What are those kids up to?

As you peek around the corner, there stand Carolina and Will thoroughly enjoying that classic preschool pastime, "playing doctor." They have shed their clothes and are busily examining each other. *Now* what do you do?!

You could react with shock and anger: *"What are you two doing? Put your clothes on right now, and don't ever do that again!"* Messages: The children have done something terribly wrong; it's bad to be naked or curious about each other's bodies. That's quite a response when these little ones were simply acting on the usual interest in bodies that children tend to have at this age. Now they're upset, ashamed and confused.

On the other hand, what if you remain unruffled (at least on the outside) and acknowledge the children's curiosity: *"Hey, you two look like you're having fun! Are you checking each other out to see how your bodies might be the same or different? I'd like you to put your clothes on while I get a picture book we can look at that explains all about bodies."* Messages: It's OK to be curious about bodies; I prefer you keep your clothes on when you're playing together; I'm willing to help you learn.

Parents react to this type of situation in a variety of ways. When choosing your response, think about the behavior from a child's point of view. Preschoolers are fascinated with bodies. It's natural for them to want to see how "yours and mine" compare. Since playing doctor is universally popular among young children, there's a good chance you'll get to address it in your own family. Think about how you want to handle it. With preparation, you can be ready with a thoughtful, positive response that feels good to you and your child.

A final note... no matter how you respond, be sure to discuss it with the other child's parent. They may or may not agree with how you handled things, but they will appreciate being informed. It gives them a chance to convey their own messages and beliefs to their child.

The "askable" parent

Being attentive to your child's sexuality education might feel like a big undertaking. Most of us have few good role models on which to base our own efforts. Yet in many ways, you are ideal for the job. You are the best person to teach the values and beliefs you hold and wish to share. You can always get help with factual information or ways to approach various issues. And certainly there are others who can make valuable contributions to your child's learning. Teachers, faith leaders, a favorite aunt or a trusted grandfather can potentially be important resources for your children as they grow. It's useful for children to have a network of caring adults in their lives who are approachable, available... who are "askable."

Here are a few tips to help you in the process:

- **Parents: Talk with one another** about the messages you want to give your child about sex.

- **Initiate conversations** about sex. Ask, *"Have you ever wondered about how you were born?"* Use picture books; visit a pregnant friend.

- **Use everyday events** as "teachable moments."

- **Answer questions as they come up.** Replies such as, *"Not now,"* and *"You don't need to know that at your age,"* teach children that it's not OK to ask... or not OK to ask *you.* You can postpone a discussion with, *"I do want to answer your question. This just isn't a good time. Can we talk after dinner?"* Then follow through!

• **Tell your child** if you're feeling awkward or uncomfortable. You can say to your child, *"This is a little hard for me to talk about, but let me try."* S/he will appreciate your honesty.

• **Answer simply and truthfully.**

• **Check for understanding and leave the door open** for further discussion. You might say things like, *"Does that answer your question?" "Does that make sense?" "Is there something else you'd like to know?" "You can always ask me."*

Learn and think about the sexual questions/behaviors that are common for children at various ages. It gives you the chance to consider and practice how you want to respond.

Here are just a few sexual issues that are typical for many young children, along with ideas for responses that are forthright, age-appropriate and honest:

Q. How do you make a baby?

A. Sometimes a mommy and daddy make a baby together. A special cell called a sperm cell from the daddy joins with a special cell called an ovum or egg inside the mommy's body. That starts a baby growing.

Q. How does the daddy give a sperm cell to the mommy?

A. There are a few ways that can happen. One way is that the sperm swim out of the daddy's penis and into the mommy's vagina. The sperm then move to the place inside the mommy's body where the ovum or egg cell is waiting. Is there more you'd like to know?

Q. Why don't girls have penises?

A. Boys and girls have a lot of the same body parts, but some of their body parts are different.

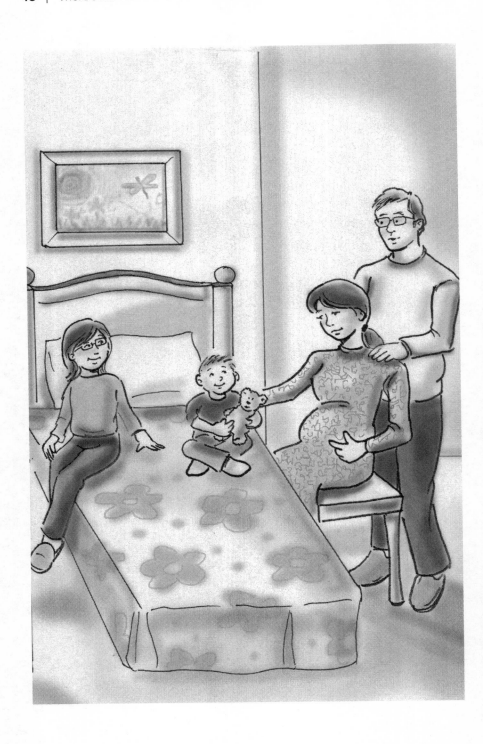

Q. *Like what?*

A. *Well, most girls have a uterus inside their bodies. This is the place where a baby grows when a person is pregnant.*

(Note: Once again, be mindful that the sexual anatomies of some males and females are not that clear-cut and typical. Respond to your child's questions in a way that also speaks to his or her experience.)

Q. *Why did grandma get mad at me for touching my penis? I was in my room like you told me.*

A. *Not all people have the same ideas or beliefs about things. Grandma thinks about this differently than we do. I'm glad that you remembered that touching your penis is something you do in private, like in your room – and not where other people can see.*

It can be tricky when parents are caught by these questions unprepared. Having a chance to reflect on them ahead of time allows you to pull your facts together and think about the beliefs that you hold and want to share with your child. Based upon those facts and beliefs, you can then shape responses you feel good about and that are accurate, affirming and reflective of your values.

Wait... haven't we already been over this?

Throughout your child's early years, you will be called upon to repeat the same "sexplanations" again and again... and yet again. Your preschooler learns by asking questions – LOTS of them! As you respond to sexual questions with patience and honesty, you're letting your child know, *"You're important to me. I am willing to take time with you,"* and *"I'm glad you asked me. This is a good topic for us to talk about."*

Children's sexual curiosity can surface at the most inopportune times: during dinner at grandma's house, on a crowded elevator, in line at the checkout stand. It helps to keep your sense of humor about it. If you're not able or willing to discuss it at that moment, let your child know it's the timing that's bad, not the question or the topic. *"I'm glad you asked me, Evan. We'll have time to talk about it on the way home."* This is far more supportive and positive than a stern, *"Evan, hush!"* or worse yet, silence.

So your child's questions cause a bit of embarrassment, or the timing's awkward. The great news is that s/he feels comfortable asking you.

If young ones aren't asking a parent about sex, it may be that they've already sensed that it's not OK to ask, or that these kinds of questions make people upset or uncomfortable. Over time they may turn elsewhere to find the answers... to friends, the Internet, experimentation. This can lead to misinformed, vulnerable youth.

Most parents want to provide (and children want to receive) information and guidance in the area of sexuality. You can make that happen!

Naked or not?

Parents often wonder about nudity in the family and how that might affect their children. Is it OK or problematic? Is there an age at which I should insist that my child – or my partner/spouse – wear clothes around the house?

While children are young, many parents have a relaxed attitude about nudity. During these early years, nudity among family members in natural situations (taking a shower, getting undressed) can provide opportunities for children to find out about body parts and physical differences between genders as well as between kids and grown-ups. It can send a message of self-acceptance and comfort with one's body. This is a healthy attitude for children to learn.

Much beyond the toddler stage, parents might find themselves questioning the appropriateness of nudity, especially with children of another gender. Some parents are uncomfortable being undressed around their children and take advantage of other ways to teach them about the wonders of human bodies. Children's picture books can be great tools.

It's important to talk with children about when and where it's OK to be naked (for example, at home with family members or when getting a checkup at the doctor's office vs. at the store or in other public places).

There's also the lesson about respecting privacy:

Q. Mommy, why can't I come into the bathroom when you're in the shower? Kai does with his mom.

A. That's something people and families get to decide for themselves, Kellen, depending on what they feel comfortable with. I like to be by myself when I shower.

One way we teach our children about respecting others' space and privacy is by being respectful of theirs. Knocking on a closed door before entering, allowing private (safe) use of the bathroom... these behaviors let your child know you appreciate his/her wish for privacy.

Often the whole question of nudity at home takes care of itself when young children begin to express their own preferences. They may not want to be seen undressed in front of others or see a parent or sibling unclothed. This is quite individual from one child to the next. Families should respect those feelings.

Some children are quite comfortable with nudity in the family, even well beyond their early years. So back to the original question: nudity at home, yes or no? There's no one answer that fits all. Trust that you have some good intuition about these sorts of issues. Take your cues from your own gut and from your child's reactions.

Speaking of privacy...

You forgot to remind Darren not to enter your bedroom without knocking if the door is closed. He woke up hearing noises coming from your room and came in to see what was going on. You've been caught in the act!

Awkward, right? It might be the ultimate challenge for parents to stay cool under such circumstances. It's hard to avoid the inclination to shout, *"What are you doing here?! Go back to your room!"* or *"I've told you, don't come into our room without knocking!"*

Through a little one's eyes and ears, sex can look and sound like fighting or like a parent is being hurt. It's important that parents remain calm and be reassuring. *"Everything's OK, sweetie. Daddy and I were playing together and loving each other. Do you need something?"*

Later, parents could follow up, and encourage their child to talk about why he came into their room in the first place, and what he was thinking or feeling when he saw them. It's good practice to help children talk about their thoughts, feelings, worries or confusion. They learn to identify and express what they're feeling, and they learn that their parents will listen and take the time to understand.

In this situation, by being open to Darren's questions, and by responding simply and honestly, his parents can both educate and reassure. Handled with understanding and love, this can be yet another teachable (although challenging) moment for imparting valuable lessons about sex.

It's good practice to help children talk about their thoughts, feelings, worries or confusion. They learn to identify and express what they're feeling, and they learn that their parents will listen and take the time to understand.

Protecting children from sexual abuse

It's easy to feel paralyzed with fear that your child could be sexually abused, and it can seem overwhelming to even broach the subject with them. Yet we know it's important that we do what we can to protect them. Here are several ways to teach and empower children without making them fearful and distrustful:

- **Impress** upon your child, *"Your body is your own, and you can say 'no' if anyone touches you in a way you don't want, don't like, or in a way that just feels uncomfortable."*

- **Talk** about the differences between good and bad touching. Ask your child to help you describe what good touch feels like. Make the point that it's pleasant and welcomed. Be concrete with examples of good touch – hugging or cuddling (as long as it is appropriate and with permission). Bad touch hurts, is uncomfortable, or just feels like it shouldn't be happening. Again, be clear with examples – being pinched, having someone touch your penis or vulva when you don't want them to, a hug that is too tight or forced on you.

- **Encourage** your child to recognize and trust that feeling in her body that says something isn't right. Help her describe the feeling she might get in her stomach, chest or elsewhere inside of her.

- **Allow** your child to decide whether s/he wants to give or get hugs and kisses. Offer affection to your youngster rather than imposing it. Substitute, *"Can I have (or give you) a hug?"* for, *"Give me a hug."* This helps your child feel a sense of control over his/her body.

- **Emphasize** that no one has the right to touch a child's genitals or to ask a child to touch his/her genitals. Explain that this includes family members. *"I want you to tell me if that ever happens."*

- **Differentiate** between "secrets" and "surprises." A surprise is something that is OK to tell at some point (like a surprise birthday present). Your child should not be told to keep secrets from you.

- **Practice** "what if" with your child: *"What if someone you didn't know asked you to help them find their lost dog? What if the baby sitter promised you more ice cream if he could touch your penis/vulva? What would you say? What would you do?"* Rehearsing exact words and actions can help your child react in uncomfortable or dangerous situations.

Awareness, communication and assertiveness serve children well. Building these strengths in your kids will promote their protection and safety.

Early Elementary
Level

Kids need to know... parents need to tell them

Most 5-year-olds have had a bit of experience in the world: interactions with family; exposure to other children, diverse families and differing beliefs; chances to view TV shows, movies, magazines, advertising. All of these things inform and influence a child's developing sense of what sexuality and relationships are all about. Everyday situations and events lend themselves to a child's sex education.

When parents dismiss their children's sexual questions and behaviors, or respond with alarm, annoyance or scolding, it implies that sexuality is bad or dirty. When they respond with delight and take these opportunities to offer loving, honest explanations, teach values and set boundaries, they help their children understand that sexuality is a wonderful part of being human. Your approach with your children affects their own awareness and skills to communicate about sex.

There's a lot of foundation building going on in these early years. When children are taught and encouraged to talk clearly and honestly about sexual issues, it benefits them in their personal relationships throughout their growing up years and beyond.

The time to begin talking with your children about sexual issues may be far earlier than you imagined... and it's never too late to start. You're not your children's *only* sex educator. You are their first and most important.

What will the neighbors think?

Or grandma and grandpa? What will they think when they hear you being so open with your children about sexual topics?

We all have our own ideas about sexuality and what information is appropriate for children. You're likely to find family members, friends, teachers and other parents whose ideas and values are very different from your own. Don't let this challenge your resolve to talk honestly with your child about sex. There's a lot to be said for children knowing they can depend on their parents to talk with them about sexual issues in a forthright, respectful way.

"But what if he goes around the neighborhood sharing this information with all his friends? Then what?" OK, that can be awkward, but so what? Let him know you're glad that you and he talk with each other about these things. Then tell him it's important to let other parents have the chance to talk with their own children in the way that feels right to them. It's not up to him to take that on.

Let's face it: Kids share information with each other about lots of topics, including sex, whether parents want them to or not. Frequently it's misinformation. If your bottom line is that children deserve quality sex education, you'll figure out how you can best make that happen in a way that is responsive to your child and respectful of others. Parents don't have to apologize for providing that education — no matter who disagrees.

What did you say?!

"Mary! Don't let me hear you say that word again!"

Mary knows certain words make daddy holler. She's not sure why. She doesn't know what the words mean... or why they're bad. What's really confusing is, why doesn't daddy holler at his friends when *they* use those words? And why does *he* say them?

Parents can be caught off guard the first time they hear their little ones utter a four-letter word they've picked up at preschool (or at home, for that matter). Before responding, it can be useful to consider why a child might be using those words. S/he could be:

- **Looking for attention.** In this case, some parents choose to ignore the initial use of such language, but step in if it continues.

- **Looking for information.** Children often use these words and have no idea what they mean. They may sense some words are shocking or provocative and are looking for confirmation. A parent could ask, *"Do you know what that word means?"* and then define it. *"Is that what you want to say?"* A response like this neutralizes the word, provides information, and demonstrates the parent's willingness to talk about sexual issues and language.

- **Expressing anger or frustration.** It's important that parents acknowledge those feelings and help the child choose different words to express them. *"You sound angry. Can you tell me what it's about? It's OK to feel angry. I just don't like the words you're using. What other words can you use to show that you're angry?"*

Certain parent responses can be counterproductive and result in continued use of offensive language. Laughing implies the behavior is cute or funny. Overreaction and harsh punishment can lead to anger and resentment. Ignoring the behavior for an extended period of time implies that it's acceptable.

As parents, we can all do well to remember that we might also want to watch our own language. "Do as I say, not as I do" doesn't cut it. Model the behaviors you want to encourage.

Lots of ways to be a family

Some families have a mom and a dad. Some have a mom. Or two moms. A guardian. Stepparents. Two dads. There is a lot of diversity — all kinds of ways to create loving families and raise healthy children.

Early on, children experience and interact with a variety of families and family structures, perhaps more so than their own parents did when they were growing up. Help your children appreciate that not all families look the same, and that each is unique and special in its own way. We enrich our conversations with children about sexuality and loving relationships when we include discussions about families that form in other ways than our own.

"Daddy, what's gay marriage? I heard them talking about it on TV."

> *We enrich our conversations with children about sexuality and loving relationships when we include discussions about families that form in other ways than our own.*

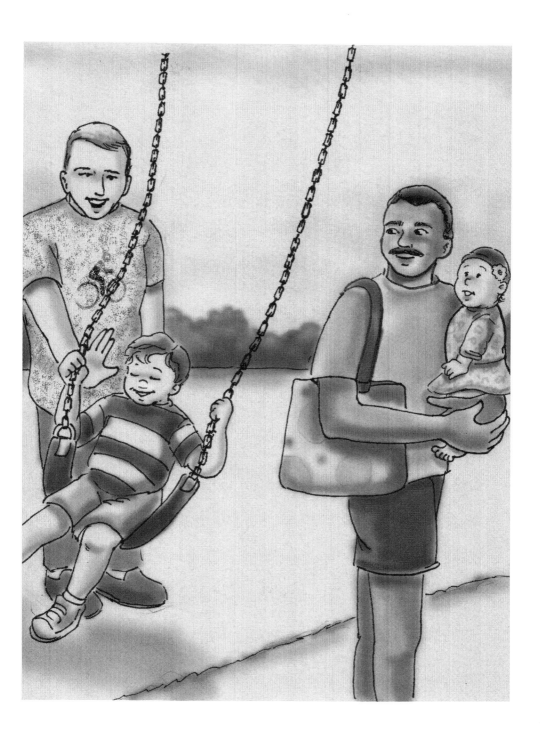

"Jamie has two mommies. She never had a daddy. How does that happen?"

"But if two men get married, can they have a baby?"

For a 5-year-old, these kinds of questions don't require answers with lengthy, graphic detail. But they do need to be answered. Remember to think about children's questions from their perspective. Take the time you need to form answers you feel good about... even if it means delaying the conversation with something like, *"Hey, that's a really good question. Thanks for asking me. I'm not sure how to answer right now, and I'd like to talk with you about it a little bit later, OK? How about after dinner?"* Find more information if you need it, and consider what else you want to convey to your child beyond the factual information.

Here's one discussion idea:

Son: *Daddy, what's gay marriage? I heard them talking about it on TV.*

Dad: *Well, that's when two men who love each other get married. Or two women who love each other get married. Just like your mom and I love each other and we're married. Does that make sense?*

Son: *But if two men get married, can they have a baby?*

Dad: *Sure. One thing they might do is adopt a baby.*

Son: *That's OK?*

Dad: *People have different ideas about that. I believe that what's most important is that children have parents who love and take care of them... whether it's two dads or two moms, a mom and a dad or just one parent. What do you think?*

Pretty basic and straightforward, right? This is just one example of how a parent might talk about questions that may feel challenging and complex at first, but in reality can be addressed in a simple, responsive and positive way.

But Scott's dad said...

As children interact and become more involved with others they will also be exposed to varying attitudes, values and expectations. It can be confusing, so it's important that parents talk about personal beliefs. For example:

Dad: *Johnny, I just got off the phone with Scott's dad. He was upset about how you and Scott were playing today.*

Johnny: *I know. He yelled at us for taking our clothes off.*

Dad: *How come you were naked? Were you running around under the sprinkler?*

Johnny: *No.*

Dad: *Oh… well, why did you need to have your clothes off?*

Johnny: *We were being doctors and doing checkups.*

Dad: *I see. And what did Scott's dad do when he saw that?*

Johnny: *He yelled at us and said it was nasty. He made us stop.*

Scott's dad was alarmed at seeing his son and another boy undressed, looking at each other and touching each other's bodies. Maybe he was worried this was "abnormal," or was upset because he believes it's not OK for kids to be naked in front of each other. His angry response left the children feeling hurt, ashamed and "nasty."

Johnny's dad believes that "playing doctor" is a common childhood experience – between children of the same and other genders. Young children are interested in bodies – how they look, feel, work – and they're particularly curious about "how yours compares to mine."

He realizes that often parents forget that a child's sexual behavior does not have the same significance it does for adults. He also respects that families have different values and beliefs about what is and isn't appropriate with regard to sexual behaviors. His concern right now is to restore Johnny's positive feelings about himself, his body, his natural curiosity and his sexuality.

Dad: *Why do you suppose Scott's dad was angry?*

Johnny: *He thought we were being nasty.*

Dad: *Do you think you were?*

Johnny: *No.*

Dad: *I don't think so either. Sounds like you and Scott were interested in finding out about bodies. That's pretty normal.*

Johnny: *Scott's dad thinks it's bad.*

Dad: *Well, he may believe it's not OK for kids to play without their clothes on. Some families feel that way. So when you're playing with Scott, be sure to respect that and keep your clothes on. Make sense?*

Johnny: *OK.*

Dad: *I have a book that shows all kinds of bodies and how they work. Let's read it together.*

Johnny just had a valuable experience with his dad and learned some important lessons from him: His dad is interested in talking with him about these issues and willing to help Johnny learn; it's normal to be curious about bodies and wonder what they look like; people have different beliefs and expectations and it's important to respect that. Underlying all of this is a positive, affirming sense about sexuality.

Good work, Dad!

A little help?

There are many resources that provide extensive information and sex education strategies that are quite good. Some dive more deeply into targeted issues that are not addressed in detail here (for example: gender identity and concerns of single parents, adoptive and blended families, and gay- and lesbian-headed families). See the Resource Section for more information, including web sites, publications and organizations. Also consider local resources such as Planned Parenthood, the health department, family counselors, your personal doctor or your faith community.

The pregnancy/childbirth conversation… kindergarten-rated

Parents are often surprised how early children begin asking where babies come from. At 3 and 4, they're mostly wondering how the baby comes out. The 5-year-old is concentrating on how that baby gets *in*.

Yes, it's an age-appropriate question. And the conversations you have about it at this age can build your children's knowledge as well as their trust that you're a good (and willing) resource.

As is often the case, it's useful to let children guide the discussion. You might ask, *"What ideas do you have about how babies are made?"* The response you get will help you decide what comes next. There are many ways this conversation can go depending on how family was created in your home. This is just one way, relevant to one type of family structure:

Parent: *A mommy's body has tiny cells called eggs. A daddy's body has tiny cells called sperm. One way a baby is made is when an egg cell and a sperm cell join together inside the mommy. That starts a baby growing.*

Child: *How does the sperm get into the mommy?*

Parent: *Sperm leave the daddy through his penis and go into the mommy's vagina. They find their way to the place in the mommy's body where the egg is.*

Child: *And then what?*

Parent: *If the egg and sperm join together, they can grow into a baby in a special place inside the mommy's body. It's called the uterus. Is there more you want to know?*

It's true that 5-year-old thinking is very literal. You might explain that the egg cell is not like a chicken egg. It doesn't have a hard shell, and it is very tiny… like the size of a dot made on a paper with a sharp pencil. Or you can go totally scientific and use the term "ovum," avoiding the possible confusion in the first place. "Sperm" rather than "seed" prevents the idea of flowers blooming in mommy's uterus. Consider using age-appropriate books on this subject to help your child understand.

You will have many opportunities to refine and add to this story as your children grow. Each positive conversation sets the stage for others to come.

When children don't ask

If your 5-year-old doesn't seem the least bit interested in sexual issues and hasn't asked any questions, initiate the conversations.

Everyday events lend themselves to talking about sexuality (a neighbor is pregnant, the hamsters are mating, etc.). Take advantage of that. You can be proactive and intentional with your child's sexuality education:

- **Read** children's picture books on topics related to bodies, babies and families. Include them in your child's collection of books and read them together.

- **Look** at family albums with photos of weddings and civil unions, pictures of mom when she was pregnant, or snapshots of the new baby being welcomed into the family.

- **Ask** your child to draw a family picture or pictures of their friends and their families. Talk about similarities and differences.

You might consider that your child has indeed been asking about sexuality — often in nonverbal ways — since birth. You may not have recognized it as such, or perhaps you or someone else has given an impression that it's not OK to ask. Whatever has or has not been going on, start something now.

Let's talk

This is it. First grade — the big time. You're delighted and proud to see your children learning and growing. You may also be a little anxious about ratcheting up the number of "outside influences" your children will now be exposed to.

First-graders are gaining a stronger sense of themselves in relation to a larger world. They begin to consider how they fit in with new friends and school acquaintances. What they see, hear and read makes an impression. It's a good time to remember the importance of having that history of trust and openness with your child — especially in the area of sexuality.

If that history isn't in place, it's not too late to start. *But do start now.* The early years are critical to helping your child develop healthy attitudes toward sexuality. And it's far easier to talk about sexuality with your children if you make it a habit while they are young. Family discussions about sex can:

- **Allow** parents to share important values.

- **Support** children in forming positive attitudes and healthy respect toward sexuality.

- **Ease** anxieties or confusion that children often have about their sexual curiosity.

- **Build** trust, understanding and support.

- **Increase** the likelihood that children will look to parents for information and guidance about these issues in the future.

Your child is launching his school career. What better gift to give him than your commitment to supporting growth and understanding in all aspects of his being – including sexuality!

OK... where do I begin???

Begin by appreciating where first-graders are at with their sexual curiosity and why some hesitate to ask about things that have to do with sex. Children have usually developed fairly perceptive "radars" by this age that alert them to topics and behaviors that adults find unacceptable or uncomfortable. So they're wary of saying or doing things that might cause trouble. The early grade school child is naturally curious about a number of sexual issues – whether that interest is verbalized or not. They wonder about:

- Where babies come from.

- Body parts and functions.

- Gender similarities and differences, roles, and expectations.

- Sexual language.

So the ball may be in your court to start the conversation. Here are some reminders:

- **Listen** to your child's questions – and be sure you understand what s/he's really asking.

- **Answer** simply and honestly.

- **Don't worry** about telling "too much, too soon." Children absorb what they are ready to, and are not overstimulated or encouraged by more detail. The real worry lies in "too little, too late."

- **Have fun with this!**

Empowering children

"Don't take candy from strangers." Remember this classic warning from your own childhood? Usually coupled with, *"Never talk to strangers,"* this rather vague precaution never quite addressed parents' deeper concerns and fears about sexual abuse.

Studies suggest that one out of every four children in this country experience some form of sexual victimization before age 17; 15% to 20% are boys. Contrary to the early warnings of our own parents, the typical child molester is *not* the stranger who entices children with candy. In fact, 70% to 80% of abusers are known to the child – and are often related.

When parents foster self-reliance and assertiveness in their children they are helping build protection from sexual abuse. But what else can be done?

First, families must abandon the idea that "it can't happen to me." Sexual abuse crosses all socioeconomic lines, religious beliefs and ethnicities. Every child should learn safety information and skills:

- Have your child use proper terms for body parts. Substitute words like "penis" and "vulva" for vague descriptors like "private parts" and "down there."

- Emphasize that your child's body is his own. No one has the right to touch him in ways he doesn't like. He has the right to say no to unwanted or uncomfortable touch.

- Let your child decide whether and when to be affectionate. Forcing hugs and kisses is unfair and lessens a child's feeling of control over her own body.

- Explain that no adult has the right to touch a child's penis (vulva, etc.) or to ask a child to touch his/her genitals. This applies to family members too (explain possible exceptions such as a parent helping a child bathe).

- Tell your child she has the right to say no to any adult who asks her to do something wrong. *"It's wrong for a grown-up to ask you to lie or steal. It's also wrong for them to touch you or ask to be touched in the ways we talked about. You should say no, then come and tell me."*

- Explain that no one should insist your child keep secrets from you. *"If someone touches your penis/vulva, and warns you not to tell me, it's likely because it was wrong for them to do that. Secrets and surprises are different. At some point you can tell people about surprises (like the present mom bought dad for his birthday)."*

- Practice "what if" with your child. *"What if the baby sitter promised you could stay up later if you touched his penis?"* *"What if a stranger came to the door while I was in the shower?"* Rehearse specific words and actions. Help your child know what to do if s/he feels threatened — where to go and names of trusted adults who can help if parents are not available.

Talking about sexual abuse isn't easy. You may worry about frightening the children, or about what to say and how to say it. Much of this anxiety stems from the discomfort people often have about discussing sexual issues in general. In addition to the basic tips offered here, there may be excellent resources available through your local Planned Parenthood, the health department, your physician's office or a sexual assault center.

No gender limitations

"That's girl *stuff,"* Marty insists when you ask him to help set the dinner table. *"Boys aren't supposed to do girl stuff."*

Cringing at what you've just heard, you think, *"Wait a minute. Where did* that *come from?"* Recently he's made several comments smacking of gender stereotyping that you dislike. What's up with that?

Old influences die hard. The school-age child has ventured into a world where they have daily experiences with others who look at the world quite differently. Historically, expectations – and *limitations* – based on gender have been a way of life in this society: One set of standards, values and behaviors considered acceptable for boys; a different set appropriate for girls. The general attitude about this is changing, yet for many, biases persist.

It's an important time to remind the 6-year-old that **goals and expectations need not be limited by gender.** Help your child appreciate that people – no matter their gender – are capable of lots of things.

As parents work to broaden their children's thinking, they may find themselves at odds with influences of the outside world. Rather than set up a "we're right, they're wrong" struggle, it's useful to approach it as "here's *another* way to look at things." In the arena of gender roles and expectations, it's empowering to children to have other ways of looking at things.

But what if...

Many parents admit they avoid talking about sexual issues with their children and assume that somewhere along the line, kids will learn what they need to know. It's likely that these very same parents *want* to be involved in their children's sexuality education... they just feel ill-prepared to do so. Fear, confusion and embarrassment are some of the barriers that get in the way. Let's take a look at a few concerns parents often express:

- *I'm worried that giving too much sexual information will cause my child to be even more curious and encourage him to experiment.* This is related to the fear of telling too much, too soon. Children's curiosity about sexuality is a natural thing. If that curiosity is ignored, denied – or worse yet, punished – they may become preoccupied with the subject and even more determined to find answers in some other way.

- *But she's only in first grade. Isn't that too young?* For lengthy, graphic detail? Of course. But not for some basic information. Your explanations can be simple, clear and factual. At the same time, leave the door open for further discussion. Remember, now is the time to establish the foundation for open communication... an environment in which your child knows it's safe and appropriate to ask questions or voice opinions.

- *I don't want to frighten or confuse my child.* Children are more concerned and confused when they only have bits and pieces of information... or misinformation. It leaves much to their imaginations, which can fabricate some rather frightening details. By first grade, your children have heard *something* about sexual issues. It's helpful when you talk with them about these topics – intentionally, honestly, and with a willingness to address any questions or worries they might have.

- *I'm not sure I have my facts straight.* That can be the *least* of your worries. If you don't know the answer, say so. Then offer to look it up. Better yet, suggest that the two of you find the answer together.

In addition to factual information, many excellent resources are available to help in the "how to" department. Check with your local Planned Parenthood, the health department, or your physician's office.

It's partly about self-esteem

It's hard to believe that first grade is almost over. What a milestone for your youngster — a full year of real school just about completed. Along with accomplishments, perhaps your first-grader has also had some disappointments and frustrations. How has s/he fared? As a whole, has the year been a joyful experience and a positive venture into the world of school?

And just what does any of this have to do with sex education? Plenty. You see, research tells us that self-esteem influences the sexual decisions and behaviors of adolescents. High self-esteem relates to an increased likelihood that choices will be positive, healthy and responsible.

The development of self-esteem during the preschool years is based largely on experiences with family. If Theyo is constantly told he's a "bad boy," he'll soon define himself as such — and act accordingly. It's important for his parent to emphasize that it's his *behavior* that's not OK (not Theyo himself).

Once in school, children are exposed to pressures, demands and expectations that reach beyond the home front. It's especially important for parents to reassure their children that a sense of worth comes from within and is not a function of appearance, being a math whiz, or getting the lead in the class play.

As with all other aspects of growth and development, children need support in feeling competent, connected and valued. Through their child raising practices, parents either foster or stifle that development. Here are some things children need from their parents:

- **Approval** – Children tend to measure their own value by their parents' approval. Recognize and praise your youngster for a good effort and a job well done.

- **Acceptance** – While recognizing your child's strengths and abilities, help him accept his weaknesses. If he acts inappropriately, be sure he understands that while you do not like the *behavior*, you still love *him*.

- **Attention** – When you show sincere interest in your child's day-to-day activities, you let her know she's important. Having a parent's *undivided attention* helps a child feel valued.

- **Achievement** – Children learn by doing and need opportunities to practice new skills. Allowing them to make decisions encourages a sense of competence and responsibility.

- **Respect** – *Children are people too.* They deserve to be treated fairly – with dignity and respect.

All of this may seem so obvious. Yet it's amazing how much good, common sense parenting gets lost in the daily bustle of family life. Consider this simply a reminder. The way children feel about themselves colors the way they live and relate to the world around them. Children who grow up feeling loved, competent and worthy are far better equipped – as adolescents and adults – to deal with the issues of life... including sexuality.

Even in elementary school kids are learning about sexuality...

They learn about it from their friends... from the media... from many other sources. Surely they deserve to learn about it from their parents.

It's probably no surprise to parents that young children take in lots of sexual messages on a regular basis. Why, remember just last weekend when you stumbled on Nick, your little second-grader, and his buddy Seth? They were having quite a chat... serious whispers punctuated by fits of giggling. All of that came to an abrupt halt the moment they spotted you! Could their conversation have been about something to do with s-e-x?

What about that movie you watched with the kids the other night? You were careful to pick something appropriate. What you hadn't counted on were the steamy previews shown before the featured show. You were more than a little uncomfortable – and unsettled – by Nick's obvious interest in them.

Your children are hearing about sexual topics whether you tell them or not. There are advantages to having you tell them.

You are the expert when it comes to framing messages within the context of your family's values. You may need a little encouragement or support to overcome your discomfort. Maybe you'd like a few tips on how to begin or how much to say. That's all fine-tuning. But the heart of the message – your values and attitudes related to sexuality – is within you.

Today's parents are raising children in a world that is markedly different from that of their youth. Intense peer and media pressures encourage sexual activity at younger ages. The realities of sexual violence, pornographic web sites, and other outside influences require that we speak to our children – at times quite explicitly – early on. Amidst all of this, the challenge is to avoid scare tactics and deliver messages that present sexuality itself in a positive light.

Ultimately, we wish for our children a sense of appreciation and high regard for their sexuality. We want them to enjoy and celebrate that very special part of their being. We want them to have self-respect and good feelings about themselves... every part of themselves, *including* their sexuality. And we want them to have accurate information. What better way to promote that vision than by providing loving, thoughtful sex education at home?

Just when you thought you had it handled...

The incidence of HIV, AIDS and other sexually transmitted diseases (STDs, which are sometimes referred to as sexually transmitted infections) raises concerns and, at times, irrational fears. We know there are Internet sites, ads, news stories, public service announcements, TV shows and more that are talking about sexual behaviors and infections, safer sex practices, condoms, dental dams, vaginal and oral sex... yikes! As parents, do you really need to discuss HIV and AIDS with your children at this age?! And if so, where do you even begin?

Remember... breathe. Your children don't need a lesson in the complexities of sexual relationships and the sexual transmission of infection. They *do*, however, need to hear from you. Even at this age.

Again, think of this as providing the foundation that will make it easier to talk about this issue in more appropriate detail later on in your child's life. It's a good time to discuss general concepts of wellness and staying healthy. Help your children appreciate that there are important habits they can form and choices they can make that promote good health — such as hand washing, dressing appropriately, eating nutritious foods, brushing their teeth, exercising, and getting plenty of rest.

You can talk basic facts about disease. For example, explain that germs can be passed from a person who is sick to a person who isn't. Some of these germs can cause a cold, flu, stomachache or chicken pox. HIV is one of those illnesses that starts with a certain type of germ that is passed to others by a person who has it in their body. The conversation can be that basic and easy.

You could ask your children if they have heard about HIV and AIDS, and if so, what they've heard. Correct any misinformation they might have picked up (or imagined). Here are a few appropriate messages about HIV and AIDS for a 5-year-old:

- AIDS is caused by a virus called HIV.

- Some viruses, including HIV, can only spread in certain ways. For example, one way HIV spreads is if blood from someone who has the virus gets into another person's body. We should always be careful and not touch another person's blood.

- We can be friends and play with people who have this virus in their bodies. HIV is *not easy* to get. We can hug them, shake hands with them, share food with them, sit next to them... there are lots of thing we can do together and not worry about getting HIV from them.

It's not too early to have this chat. Find out if and how teachers are talking with your children about these issues. Take a look at the National Health Education Standards on the Centers for Disease Control and Prevention web site – www. cdc.gov/healthyyouth/sher/standards. These standards provide a framework for school-based education to promote and support healthy behaviors for students in all grade levels, Pre-K through grade 12. You will notice that the standards for pre-kindergarten through early elementary level include, among other things, "Identify that healthy behaviors impact health," and "Describe ways to prevent communicable diseases."

Your discussions at home can build on information your children are learning in school.

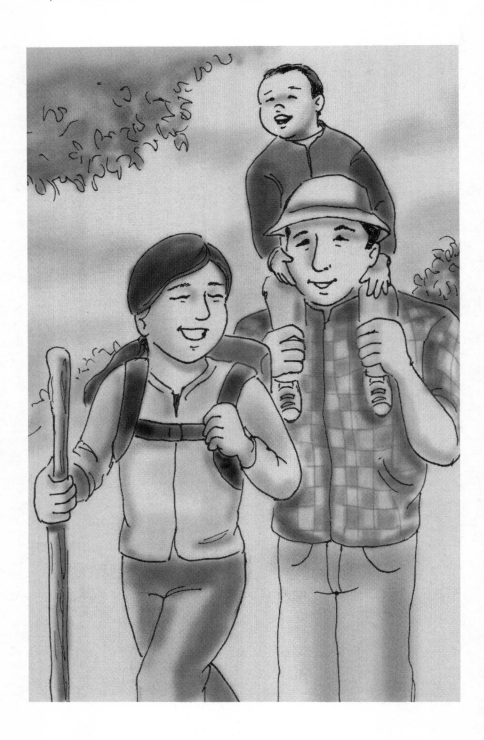

You thought *that* was hard
– wait until you try *this*...

Remember the days when your child was a preschooler and showed great interest in how babies are made? At times you may have wondered if that interest was more like preoccupation. In reality, your youngster was just naturally and appropriately curious about a fascinating subject.

As a second-grader, your child might be no less fascinated by the baby-making process (although s/he is less likely to blurt out the question in a crowded elevator... maybe). Don't assume that your earlier discussions have taken care of this topic. It's important for parents to revisit this and other sexuality topics at various times throughout their children's lives to clarify, reinforce and expand on age-appropriate information and messages.

At this age children have some difficulty grasping the idea of intercourse. Even more confusing to them is why anyone would want to *do* that. Talking about sex in the context of making babies is really pretty straightforward. It should be brief and accurate... and yes, it's appropriate at this age.

On the other hand, the thought of helping your child realize that people engage in sexual intimacy for pleasure may stop you dead in your tracks. Is *that* OK to talk about? Sure. It's important – and only fair – that children learn about this aspect of sexuality. Parents can have that conversation within a framework of love and values.

There are ample opportunities to bring up the subject of intercourse. Perhaps a neighbor is pregnant, you've just dug out your child's baby pictures, or there's a special about pregnancy and childbirth on TV. These "teachable moments" offer springboards for discussions that might go something like this:

Dad: *I'll never forget the day we told you that mom was having another baby. You were about 4 – and so excited! You had a million questions about how babies are made.*

Son: *Did you tell me?*

Dad: *We did! We explained that babies are made when two special cells join together. One of those cells, called a sperm cell, comes from the man's body. The other cell, called an ovum or egg cell, is made by the woman's body.*

Son: *How do the cells come together?*

Dad: *One way that can happen is when a man and woman want to be very close with each other in a special, loving way. The man puts his penis into the woman's vagina. That's called sexual intercourse. Sperm cells then travel out of the man's body through his penis and into the woman's body where the egg cell is.*

Son: *So people do that when they want a baby?*

Dad: *Sometimes, yes. But that's not the only reason. People also have intercourse to share a loving, pleasurable experience with each other… even when they're not trying to have a baby. It may be hard for you to understand – and that's OK. Intercourse is not for children to do. It's a special experience for adults.*

*]]]]*There are all kinds of directions a conversation like this can take. Children can learn that babies come into families in other ways as well. For instance, some children are adopted.

There are also cases in which parents need medical help to get pregnant or are in a relationship with someone of the same gender. There are people who donate egg cells and sperm cells to help in these cases. The research tells us that it is beneficial for children to learn if any of these circumstances apply to their lives. And yes, it's appropriate information for this age. Again, let your child guide you in the conversation and leave the door open for more discussion.

At some point in the not too distant future, you will want to begin discussing this issue in a much larger context: responsibilities and potential risks with sexual intimacy, making decisions about sexual behaviors and relationships, pregnancy, etc. Open and loving communication with your second-grader now helps you pave the way.

Building filters

Every day, media messages filled with sexual references, innuendoes and behaviors assault the senses. The Internet is a treasure trove of information... and a potential minefield. What's a parent to do? Demand censorship? Isolate the kids? Install screening devices and Internet filters to protect our children from online materials we find offensive?

While parents can and need to set clear boundaries with children around their media use, it's unrealistic to think we will fully prevent their exposure to sexual messages that don't align with our values or beliefs. We *can,* however, monitor what children listen to, watch, read and Google. We can listen, watch, read and search the Internet *with* them — then discuss what we find as a family. This teaches children to manage the barrage of messages.

Use all forms of media to your advantage. This offers wonderful discussion starters! Call attention to sexual messages in programs, ads, music, web sites, etc. Ask your children how they feel about them, and share your own values regarding the messages. For better and for worse, the media "teaches" young people about a broad spectrum of sexuality-related issues: relationships, stereotypes, gender, etc. Make a point to follow up and talk about them.

By helping young children recognize, examine and talk about media messages, parents teach them to develop critical viewing skills. This not only equips children with their own personal "filters" through which to process the messages, it also provides opportunities to strengthen family communication about sex.

More than meets the eye

When you think about sex education, what topics come to mind? Anatomy... having sex... pregnancy? What else? The mechanics of sex and the plumbing (some call it the "organ recital") are but a *fraction* of the subject.

Let's consider *sexuality* education in more comprehensive terms. It includes all of the above, as well as issues like body image, gender identity, self-esteem, love, sexual orientation, relationships, respect for self and others, values, decision-making, and much more. There are many facets to human sexuality that go well beyond body parts and what we do with them.

Parents, you are communicating with your children about *sexuality* issues in verbal and nonverbal ways. While doing so, you provide your children with the bricks and mortar for their own sexual attitudes, beliefs and behaviors.

Your second-grader has been curious about and learned a lot about sexuality over the last eight years, whether you've taken an active, positive role or not. Your responses (or lack of) to questions about "plumbing;" the modeling that happens in the relationship between you and your partner; the sharing of values, biases or judgments; the experiences that help your child feel valued and respected... all these things and more contribute to your youngster's *sexuality* education. Think about how you can make this learning an intentional and positive experience.

You're not alone

Many parents say they have a harder time discussing the emotions, values and other "intangibles" of sexuality with their children than they do talking about the mechanics. It may be helpful to see and hear some ways to go about dealing with the intangibles. For books and web sites, check out the Resource Section. Beyond books, what other assistance is available — something with a more personal touch?

- **Community schools and colleges** frequently offer parenting classes that address sexuality education.

- **Pediatricians, family counselors and members of the clergy** may also provide valuable insights.

- **Your child's school or the local school district office** may have suggestions on programs available for parents.

- **Your local Planned Parenthood** is an excellent source of educational programs and materials.

Consider forming a parent group in which several of you can share experiences, concerns, ideas and strategies. It helps to know how others are working on the same issues!

You did *what?!?!?!*

The note from Owen's teacher left you speechless. It seems your third-grader and some of his buddies were caught poring over an adult magazine — lots of pictures of nude women in suggestive poses — brought to school by an older boy.

"This must be one of those 'teachable moments' I keep hearing about," you say to yourself. But at this point, you're surprised, angry... maybe a mixture of emotions you haven't quite sorted out yet.

Well, there's a good starting point: Take time to sort out what you're feeling and why. That will help you figure out how to best address this incident with your son. Rather than responding on the fly (which has the potential of being a less thoughtful and positive interaction), let Owen know you need to think about this before the two of you talk.

You may decide you're feeling embarrassed by Owen's behavior (*"What must his teacher think of me? Maybe she thinks we have those kinds of magazines around our house!"*); angry (*"How could Owen look at that trash!"*); betrayed or hurt (*"I've always taught Owen to be respectful of sexuality and of women. Then he turns around and does something like this?!"*).

Once you've identified how and why you feel as you do, take a moment to consider why Owen might have been interested in such a magazine. Of course, the way to do this would be to ask him. In fact, be sure you do that. Not only will it give *him* a chance to explain, it will likely provide a good opening for some frank conversation about sexual issues.

But for now, consider a few possibilities: Owen was curious to see what female bodies look like; he wanted to go along with his friends; it was tempting to do something "forbidden;" or all of the above.

You realize that it isn't at all uncommon for children to sneak a look at adult magazines out of curiosity. Harsh (over)reaction from parents can leave them feeling embarrassed, guilty or ashamed about what is a normal sexual curiosity... yes, even at this age.

It's actually quite useful that third-graders still have a fascination with the human body. There's still time to have good conversations with them about the topic before they reach that fairly common phase of being uncomfortable or shy about their own bodies. While he's still in this pre-pubescent time of his life, it will be helpful and reassuring for Owen to learn about bodies – of all genders – at various stages of development. Please don't hesitate to use one of the many educational books available on this topic. Read it with him, explaining things like how bodies look and function, how anatomy is similar or different from one person to the next, and how bodies change during puberty.

Along with this, you want Owen to know how you feel about magazines that show people or sexuality in a way you think is disrespectful.

You're glad that you took the time to size up the situation, put it in perspective, and avoid a knee-jerk interaction with your child that you could later regret. Such responses can be more damaging than the original behavior itself.

You now have a clear sense of what you want Owen to learn from all of this, and how you want to present your message to him.

"Come on Owen, let's talk."

Tell me about...

It's not unusual for third-graders to be hesitant to ask questions about sexual issues. It isn't from lack of interest. Third-graders have a lot unanswered — typically unasked — questions. But often they've learned that the subject of sex is uncomfortable or even off-limits. A few disapproving looks or shocked, flustered or dismissive reactions can be all it takes to drive that message home.

Maybe you're feeling good that you have encouraged and supported open communication about lots of issues in your family, including sex. Remember, though, that the experiences your child has in the world beyond his family also inform and shape how he thinks about things. Societal attitudes about sexuality are often loaded with embarrassment, concern, shame, fear, etc. So you may find yourself needing to prod a bit more to get the conversation flowing with your child. You don't need to force the issue — but do initiate discussions and continue to remind your child that you're eager and willing to talk.

Here are some typical third grade questions (and ideas for age-appropriate responses) that are often left unshared between parent and child:

Q. How old do you have to be to have a baby?

A. Once a girl gets her first period, that's usually a sign that her body is able to *get pregnant. Some girls begin their periods as young as 10 or 11. Just because she is old enough to become pregnant doesn't mean it's a good idea or that she's ready to be a mother. Being a parent is a big job. It's best for girls to wait until they're grown up before they have babies.*

(This answer assumes that there has already been some conversation about periods... if not, the following is a likely question):

Q. *What's a period?*

A. *(It helps to have a simple picture of the female reproductive system handy to explain this one.) About once a month, inside a woman's body in the place called the uterus, a layer of blood and tissue grows. It forms a soft cushion that's needed if the woman gets pregnant. That cushion is an important part of helping the baby grow. But if the woman doesn't become pregnant, the cushion of blood and tissue isn't needed and passes out of her body through the vagina. That's called having a period.*

Q. *How old does a boy have to be before he's a dad?*

A. *As soon as a boy's body begins to make cells called sperm, he can cause a pregnancy. Some boys are producing sperm at age 13 or 14. Just because he has cells to help make a baby doesn't mean it's a good idea or that he's ready to be a dad.* (Again, having a picture of the male reproductive system is useful.)

Q. *When will my breasts grow?*

A. *Different people develop at different times. You're getting closer to the age when your body will begin changing... including your breasts getting bigger. I was about 12 when I started developing. Maybe you'll take after me.*

Q. *Do boys have periods?*

A. No. Remember that a period is the shedding of the blood and tissue that grows inside a woman's uterus.

(Note: Parents can broaden the conversation beyond simply male/female to acknowledge and affirm those who have an atypical sexual anatomy or who express a gender identity that differs from their physical appearance or biological makeup (see Resource Section). At this age, you can say something quite simple, such as "... and not all bodies fit into just one category, male or female. Not all bodies experience the same things. Each body is special and unique. There are lots of varieties, all wonderful in their own way.")

Q. Why is my penis so small?

A. Bodies are all different and all special. That's true about penises too! People grow in their own way and in their own time. Your penis is just the right size for you. As you get older and start developing, all parts of your body will grow... including your penis.

Q. My body is the same size as Max's body, but my penis looks really different than his.

A. Well, for one thing, Max is circumcised. That means when he was born, the flap of skin that covered the tip of his penis was taken off. Some families choose to do that for religious or other reasons. You still have that flap of skin on the tip of your penis. So you are not circumcised. Either way – circumcised or not – is normal. Are you wondering about any other ways your penis might look different?

Q. Byron's sister is having a baby and she's not even married. How can that happen?

A. Here's one way that might happen: If a man and woman have sexual intercourse, whether they're married or not, the woman might get pregnant. I wanted to be married before I had you and your brother. For me, that's the best way to raise my family, but people have different beliefs about that.

Q. *Kelsey got in trouble for saying f—k. Why's it so bad?*

A. *That's a slang word that means sexual intercourse. It's often said in anger or to hurt someone. Knowing that, can you understand why Kelsey might have gotten in trouble for using that word?*

> *Children can be pretty resourceful. If they really want answers to these questions, yet presume they can't ask a parent, they'll find other ways to satisfy their curiosity. Some of the ways may be useless. Or inappropriate. Or harmful.*

Children can be pretty resourceful. If they really want answers to these questions, yet presume they can't ask a parent, they'll find other ways to satisfy their curiosity. Some of the ways may be useless. Or inappropriate. Or harmful.

Keep talking with your kids.

Let's get ready for change

You might be thinking, *"My child's only in third grade, so puberty is quite a way off. When s/he starts to develop, then we'll talk."*

What's challenging about this approach is that it overlooks the value of preparing children for the experiences of puberty ahead of time. Having conversations about puberty well in advance allows them the benefit of knowing what to expect, and the opportunity to hash out questions or worries about the process, before it even begins.

Puberty is not something that happens overnight – or even within a few months or years. It's a process of change that occurs over a period of three to five years or more, with the preliminaries beginning as early as age 8 for some girls and age 10 for some boys. It's not too early to start discussing this issue in a positive, reassuring and age-appropriate way with your third-grader.

At this stage, the bottom line for children is to know that each person develops at their own rate. Without that basic information, children spend a lot of time worrying that "there's something wrong with me," especially if they are the early or late bloomer in their class. You can help your kids avoid that kind of anxiety.

It's important that children understand development for both males and females. After all, where is it written that only girls need to know about menstruation, or only boys get to learn about wet dreams? Since males and females interact with each other throughout the course of their lifetimes, it makes good sense for them to appreciate how each others' bodies work. Again, remember that children with uncharacteristic sexual anatomy need their parents to help them understand how their puberty experience may be different for them.

Since some children can be modest – or possibly quite shy about their bodies (although this is certainly not true for all) – there can be some reluctance to talk about development and puberty. A gentle way to encourage the conversation could include digging out pictures of your youngster at various ages, from birth to present day. Comment enthusiastically about "how much you've grown and developed over the last nine years!" Explain that there are many changes yet to come – changes that, when anticipated and understood, can be exciting and positive.

Parents can also encourage discussion by sharing what it was like for *them*… and the feelings, thoughts and experiences they had during their early years of puberty. Besides building trust and connection, this sharing can be a source of great relief to your child, who suddenly realizes, *"I'm not the only one who's ever gone through this or felt this way!"*

Puberty can be exciting and scary – *at the same time!* It is wise and thoughtful to support your child – well ahead of time – in getting ready for that adventure.

Decisions... decisions...

Sexuality education is more than just teaching sexual facts. In addition to accurate information, children need to learn skills that can help them appreciate and manage this aspect of life.

Decision-making is one of those important skills. It's not something people learn to be good at overnight. Your third-grader has made lots of decisions up to this point: who to be buddies with at school, what books to read, what games to play on the Internet, etc. At times decisions can be hasty or shaped by others who have some influence.

As children mature, life issues become more complex, decisions more involved, and outside influences even more intense. Wise parents provide many opportunities for their children to make – and learn from – choices at an early age, when the stakes are relatively minor. It's important to practice the skill of decision-making.

Young people develop confidence and life experience when they're allowed to make their own decisions. Give your child appropriate chances to do so. Certainly a third-grader can choose what to wear to school, how to spend the birthday money grandma sent, or where the family might go for a Saturday outing.

Here are a few ways parents can help their children learn good decision-making skills:

- **Help** them gather information and weigh options when making a decision.

- **Teach** them that decisions have consequences. Ask them to talk about and consider possible outcomes of each option.

- **Talk through** "what if." *"What if you decided not to study for your math test?" "What if you go out for gymnastics instead of basketball?" "What if a friend wanted you to take a snack from the store without paying?"*

- **Accept** children's decisions as long as they are within reason and not harmful. Understand they're making choices based on personal preference and taste. The decision may not be what their parent would have selected.

- **Set limits** for decision-making. If your child decides on something clearly inappropriate or dangerous, explain why you cannot accept that choice.

- **Circle back**. If the outcome of a decision doesn't turn out well, ask children what – if anything – they might have done differently. Help children learn from the experience of making decisions… those that end well and those that don't.

These early decision-making opportunities and lessons set a good foundation for young people as they enter the teen years and begin looking at choices about their relationships, sexual behaviors and health.

Tempted to think that it will be a long time before your youngster has to worry about *those kinds of decisions?* Consider that media/peer influence and pressure hit hard – and early – these days. In any case, the skill of decision-making takes time to foster and refine. It also takes practice. Help your child practice *now* – when the issues are not so vital. Begin now, and your child will be well prepared when the time comes for those kinds of decisions.

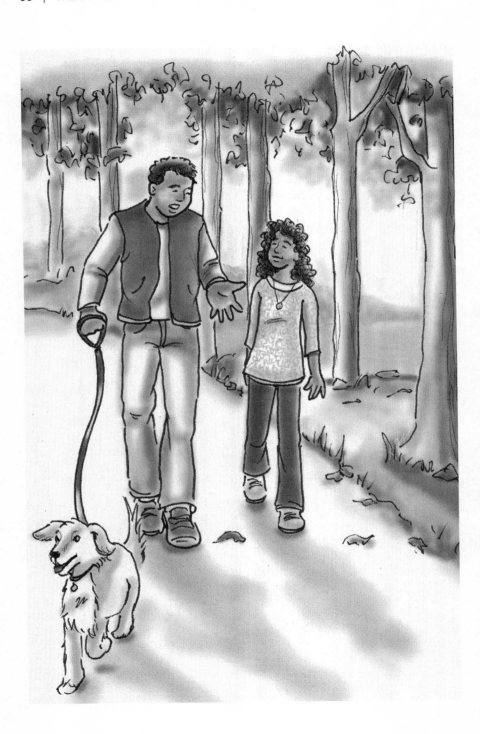

Later Elementary
Level

Family affair

Where is it written that sex education is mom's job? Or that dads should talk to the boys and moms to the girls? What about families with two moms or two dads? What about single parent homes? No matter the family structure, open communication about sexuality is the family's job. Along with information and family values, parents offer personal perspectives that are informed by their own gender identities, traditions, experiences and more.

Children will be relating to people of all genders throughout their lives. It's important that they learn about each other. Boys deserve to know about female anatomy and function, along with perspectives that may be different from their own. Girls deserve to learn about males. A parent or trusted adult of the other gender is an important resource.

(Note: For some people, the male/female distinction is not that clear-cut or exact. There are children and adults who self-identify somewhere along a continuum of being male or female – and some who identify as neither. Have discussions with young people about the variety that can exist around gender identity... again, for the purpose of understanding and appreciating themselves and others.)

This isn't to detract from the value of father-son and mother-daughter talks. On the contrary, those conversations are special times shared between a parent and child. But for men with daughters, realize that you're a valuable resource with much to contribute toward your daughters' sexuality education... just as women have much to contribute to their sons' education and awareness. So let's make sex education a family affair.

HIV and AIDS: What's age-appropriate information at this age?

The Centers for Disease Control and Prevention estimate that 50,000 new HIV infections happen each year in the United States. More than a million people aged 13 and older are living with HIV infection in the U.S. Of these, about 18% have not yet been diagnosed. While we've made tremendous advancements in HIV and AIDS research, there is still no vaccine or medication that prevents HIV infection or cures AIDS. The best protection you can offer your child is knowledge.

Your child has heard a lot about AIDS. Hopefully it's been addressed at some level in health class at school – but to what extent? Is it enough? Chances are also good that your child has heard a fair amount of misinformation and rumors about HIV and AIDS.

It's important for parents to be involved in this conversation.

Certainly by this age, children should understand that AIDS is a serious illness caused by a virus that can be passed from person to person. Reassure them that people do not become infected through casual contact (such as hugging, sharing food, or sitting next to an HIV-positive person); rather, the virus is spread through specific activities.

During the later elementary and early middle school years (9 to 12 years old), be ready to give your child more detailed information about HIV – how it spreads and how it can be prevented. Children should understand that:

- When people are infected with HIV, the virus is found in certain body fluids such as blood, semen, vaginal fluids and breast milk.

- You cannot tell whether someone has HIV simply by looking at them.

- The virus can spread if a person has unprotected sex with someone who is infected.

- HIV can also be transmitted when sharing needles with an infected person. This includes needles used to inject drugs, steroids or vitamins. Any activity that might expose someone to another person's blood can increase their risk for a number of infections.

- People can protect themselves by not having sex and not sharing needles.

- If people are having sex, using *latex* protection (condoms and dental dams) can reduce the risk of HIV transmission.

Feeling overwhelmed? There's so much sexuality information to share with your child... maybe you're not even sure of all the facts yourself! Not to worry. There are many excellent books, web sites and other resources that can help you with information, strategies and more. Check out the Resource Section at the end of this guide.

That special touch

The physical changes and sexual development that take place during the puberty years can cause a bit of anxiety and awkwardness for both children and parents. Feeling unsure about the "right" thing to do, some parents back off on the physical touch and affection they so freely gave when their children were younger.

When kids go through puberty, it can be a time of great shyness or discomfort about their physical form. Their bodies experience furious changes in size and shape. Emotions and moods can skyrocket and then plummet – all in the course of a few hours. Along with paying more attention to what their peers think, there are the appropriate signs of wanting to start detaching from their parents.

In many families, this is the stage in their children's development when parents – especially parents of the other gender – assume a "hands-off" policy when it comes to showing affection through physical touch. It can make a tough time even more confusing.

As children get older, they set up their own hands off policy. It's somewhat erratic and unpredictable. On the one hand, they might flinch at or otherwise resist a parent's attempt to hug or kiss them (especially around others). On the other hand, there are times when kids *ache* for that very thing, but don't – or *won't* – ask. Parents are expected to somehow just sense this and respond correctly.

Despite closer ties with peers and outside activities, children need to feel secure in their parents' love and acceptance. They need support and reassurance that reminds them, *"You're OK."* Let your children know you still enjoy giving and getting hugs and kisses – and that you respect their right to accept, refuse and change their minds!

All that being said, in some families and with some individuals, physical affection has never been the preferred way of showing care and support. Whatever the practice has been in your family, don't assume you have to change it up simply because your children are getting older.

Talk with them about your own uncertainty or discomfort. Encourage them to share their feelings and preferences. Decide together how to handle this "touchy" issue. Rather than automatically assuming what kids want and when, why not ask them?!

Dealing with peer pressure

Are you starting to think that your influence with your child is waning… that their peers have more clout, especially when it comes to certain issues? While there may be some truth to that, don't underestimate the value of the influence you *do* have.

For example:

According to With One Voice, a 2012 national survey conducted by The National Campaign to Prevent Teen and Unplanned Pregnancy, teens say their parents have the most influence on their decisions about sex — more than their friends, the media, their teachers or popular culture. The survey also found that nearly nine in 10 respondents (87%) felt it would be much easier for teens to delay sex and avoid pregnancy if they could have more open, honest conversations with their parents about these issues.

Surprised? Young people do want to hear from their parents, even though it doesn't always seem that way.

Young people do want to hear from their parents, even though it doesn't always seem that way. They are listening. And they are watching how you act in your own life and in your own relationships.

They are listening. And they *are watching* how you act in your own life and in your own relationships. They take all this in and learn from it. Are they learning what you would hope?

It's a sign of normal, healthy development that during the later elementary school years, young people begin increasing their separation from parents, testing their wings, becoming more independent. This is a good thing, and it can also feel scary. The world is a different place than when you were 10. Today's young people experience pressures that you probably didn't confront until much later. Drugs, alcohol, sex, violence... elementary school youth grapple with adult issues and decisions.

It's not enough to tell your child, *"Don't!"* Sometimes the need to belong and be accepted by their peer group is powerful enough that kids break the rules. It is helpful to your child when you:

- **Acknowledge** how tough it can be to go against the group.

- **Help** them recognize what peer pressure looks like – the subtle and obvious forms.

- **Share** your own experiences with peer pressure. Talk about how you dealt with different situations. Share your failures as well as your successes.

- **Practice** "what if." Brainstorm ways to respond to various scenarios. Help them analyze potential outcomes of various choices.

- **Encourage** them to come to you if they feel pressured and unsure of what to do. Offer to be their "out," their "excuse" if they need one. Kids will sometimes look to parents to say no to get them off the hook with their friends.

- **Reassure** them that even if they get into trouble, you will always be there. You may be upset, and you may even yell, but you will always be there for them and will always love them. No matter what.

Peer pressure isn't just a childhood issue. It affects young and old alike. Skills you teach your children *now* will serve them throughout their lives.

What's happening to me?

You're not the only one noticing your youngster's growth and development. S/he has too — maybe with more concern and embarrassment than enthusiasm. In fact, there have been quite a few experiences lately that have been... well... just different. Like feeling attracted to someone in more than just a friendship way. Like people talking or teasing about boyfriends and girlfriends. Things are definitely changing. And s/he's not at all sure how s/he feels about it.

While exciting, the newness is also scary. This can be a time of such privacy and shyness about change for children that they often hold their worries about, *"Is this normal?"* or *"Am I normal?"* deep within.

Menstruation and first ejaculation are often seen as landmarks that signal puberty has arrived! But in reality, puberty is a stage of life marked by a series of events — a process that unfolds over the course of several years. Menstruation and first ejaculation actually occur *later* in the process. Yet for some reason, they're seen as markers — perhaps because they're such obvious signs of growing up.

At any rate, helping your child understand the time frame of puberty can serve to ease classic fears like, *"Why am I growing so much faster than my friends?" "How come my friends are growing and I'm not?" "When will I get my period?" "What's wrong with me?"*

Young people without much information about developmental changes can be anxious and worried about these issues. Surely you know what that's like from your growing up years. Do you recall thinking later, *"If only someone had explained what was going on with me. I could have handled it much better!"* As a parent, you can be that someone for your own child.

Since we sometimes assume that children know more about their bodies than they actually do, a good rule is to explain everything... even that which seems most obvious. That way you're likely to cover many of the unspoken concerns and questions. One of the most useful pieces of information you can share with your child is a rundown of the puberty chain of events. While it's true that children will develop at different times and rates, the sequence of events is somewhat predictable. Learning about this is so much more helpful than merely having a parent say, *"Don't worry, honey. You'll grow."*

Young people need solid information about developmental changes that happen during puberty... and not just those specific to their own gender. Having a sense of this well in advance can help lessen anxiety they might be having. Reassure youngsters that each person has his or her own time clock. The body develops when it's ready... some begin early, others later. Even if they're not satisfied with their own development schedules, children are relieved to hear that what they're experiencing is normal for them.

General order for girls:

1. Breast budding (between ages 8 and 13, on average).

2. Hips broaden.

3. Straight pubic hair.

4. Growth spurt.

5. Pubic hair becomes curly and thicker.

6. Menstruation (about two years after start of breast development).

7. Underarm hair.

General order for boys:

1. Growth of testicles and scrotum (between ages 10 and 13, on average).

2. Straight pubic hair.

3. Early voice change.

4. First ejaculation (about one year after the growth of the testicles).

5. Pubic hair becomes curly and thicker.

6. Growth spurt.

7. Underarm hair.

8. Significant voice change.

9. Beard develops.

This is just a *very* general guideline. Some young people will experience a slightly different sequence of changes, or steps that overlap. Some young people have biological conditions that cause their gender or sexual characteristics to be less clear-cut than "male" or "female." In any case, please have the conversations that make sense for your own child's situation and experience.

Of course, puberty involves more than just physical changes. Emerging sexual feelings, emotions, relationships and stresses are all parts of the picture. Children often have mixed feelings about growing up and need reassurance that such feelings are perfectly normal.

Encourage them to talk about how they feel about growing and changing. Ask what they're looking forward to and what they're nervous about. Share *your* stories about puberty. Kids love being in on their parents' lives. It helps build connection and trust. It also reassures children that their folks really do understand what they're going through.

The Female Reproduction System

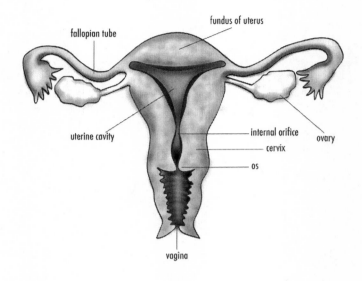

The Male Reproduction System

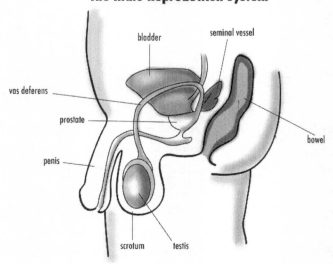

If your child is shy or genuinely uncomfortable talking about this, acknowledge it. You could say, *"If you feel awkward talking about this with me, I get it. I'm feeling a little awkward too. Maybe we can help each other get past that."*

If s/he's reluctant to talk, don't force it. Look for other opportunities to bring up the subject. There are many ways to share important information with your child. Get some of the helpful books written specifically for young people during this stage of life (see Resource Section). Leave them around the house where your child is sure to find them. (You should read them too. A puberty refresher can provide you with facts you've long since forgotten… or perhaps never knew!) There are terrific web sites such as www.kidshealth.org that cover a wide range of health-related issues in fun and interesting ways. Sometimes these resources can help young people open up a bit more to the conversation. At the very least, they will be getting good information.

Above all, be available and willing to talk. Don't be pushy, or make a big deal of it… simply seize on those opportunities that allow the topic of sexuality to come up. Puberty is a lengthy process, unfolding over the course of several years. Why not do all you can to ease the transition? Your child will not be the only one who benefits!

What I want to know is...

What causes twins? Do boys have periods? Can you get pregnant if you haven't gotten your period? What if a guy uses up all his sperm? How does birth control work? What's a wet dream? How does sex give you AIDS? How old are you supposed to be before you start having sex? How do two guys have sex? How do lesbians have babies?

These questions were asked by a typical group of fifth-graders during their human growth and development class. Some questions may surprise you because they seem so basic. You're thinking, *"Surely fifth-graders know that!"* Others shock you. *"Really? They asked about that — in fifth grade?!"*

You'd be amazed how much people this age have heard about sex. You might also be surprised both by how *little* and how *much* they really know. It can put parents in an awkward spot. On the one hand, they often assume (incorrectly) that children understand far more than they actually do. Consequently, many overlook the basics of sexuality, assuming that, *"Kids get this in health class, don't they?"* On the other hand, parents may hold back on more explicit sexual issues, assuming (again, often incorrectly), *"That's beyond what a fifth-grader needs to know."*

Truth? Young people are bombarded with sexual messages from every possible source. These messages can be inaccurate, perhaps irresponsible, even exploitative; a few may be factual and useful. Do these messages contain the values you want your child to learn? Is it any wonder 10-year-olds ask both sexually simplistic AND explicit questions?

While you might need to brush up on the facts, the best way to ensure the quality of your child's sex education is to be a main provider of that education. That's not to suggest sex education doesn't also belong in schools. On the contrary, there are a number of excellent school-based programs. For some young people, these programs are their only source of accurate information. Ideally, school-based sex education happens in combination with — not in place of — parent-child communication about sex.

Faith communities can also play an important role in educating young people about sexuality. For example, the Our Whole Lives (OWL) curriculum is a series of sexuality education programs for children in kindergarten through grade 12. Developed by the United Church of Christ and the Unitarian Universalist Association, OWL provides accurate, age-appropriate information while helping learners clarify their values, build interpersonal skills, and understand the spiritual, emotional and social aspects of sexuality. This curriculum is taught in congregations around the country and is readily adaptable to the needs of many faith traditions.

Don't be discouraged if you've not had much discussion about sexual issues with your child. It's never too late to begin. Perhaps your reluctance was due to awkwardness, uncertainty or fear – or maybe you were simply unaware of the need. Whatever the reason, you might begin your conversation by acknowledging that to your child... something like, *"You know, talking with you about sex, relationships and growing up has always been a bit tough for me. I do think it's important. I'd like to hear your concerns and thoughts, and try to answer questions you have. I'd also like to help you understand my beliefs and values."*

This doesn't have to be formal. In fact, the less formal the better... you'll both feel more comfortable. Take advantage of everyday "teachable moments." Mention an article or blog you read about teen pregnancy, a news report on HIV and AIDS, or a class assignment about reproductive anatomy. These are great discussion starters. If your child hasn't shown signs of puberty, chances are some of her peers have. That's a perfect subject to talk about since young people typically have a lot of questions and worries about it.

There are all kinds of opportunities to discuss topics related to sexually, if only you're open to them. And remember to raise those issues you assumed were too advanced. It's clear from the questions in the human growth and development class: Children have bits and pieces of hearsay, a lot of confusion, and plenty of curiosity about sex. Consider explaining what you think they want to know – and *more.*

Urges and surges

The physical and emotional changes of puberty are pretty obvious to parents. But the sexual feelings, urges and fantasies your child may be having... they're usually kept hidden and unspoken. They can leave young people feeling confused, embarrassed or ashamed (*"Is this supposed to happen?" "Is it wrong for me to be feeling this way?"*).

Reassure your child that these new and intense sexual feelings are normal, healthy, and part of the wonder and excitement of growing up! Masturbation, crushes on peers of the other gender (and the *same* gender), interesting physical responses that are different than any they've had before… they're all typical and part of the process. And the experiences can be very different from person to person.

If you haven't built a foundation on which to discuss sexual feelings, it makes it tougher… but not impossible. Here are some things you might say to your child to break the ice:

- *"I remember being 11 and having a lot of new feelings and urges. I wasn't sure what to make of them. I know a lot of my friends felt the same way, but unfortunately, no one ever talked about it. It made it really hard for me."*

- *"When I was in fifth grade, I was madly in love with a seventh grade boy. My heart would pound whenever I saw him. I had never felt anything like it. Have you ever had that happen?"*

- *"When I was your age I didn't think I could talk with my parents about sex, but I had lots of questions. How can I help you feel comfortable talking with me about these issues?"*

Facts, not fears

As sexual feelings emerge, some young people begin wondering (perhaps *worrying*) about sexual orientation. How can you tell if you're gay or lesbian? What causes it? If you masturbate, does it mean you're gay? If you have sexual thoughts about people of the same gender, does that mean you're gay?

Part of growing up is figuring out who you are. It can take a long time to do that, so questioning, exploring and experimenting are very much part of the process. Same-gender friends may check each other out, partly in an effort to validate their own

Part of growing up is figuring out who you are. It can take a long time to do that, so questioning, exploring and experimenting are very much part of the process.

development, or they might have sexual fantasies that include one another. Young people can develop crushes on same-gender peers, teachers, coaches, celebrities. It's painfully common for people who are gay, lesbian or gender nonconforming to be the target of hurtful remarks and bullying. Top all this off with a lack of information or no one to talk to about these things... is it really any wonder that many young people feel anxious, confused or afraid, no matter what their sexual orientation or gender identity?

There have been welcome changes in our culture around these topics. People who are gay or lesbian can now serve openly in the military. We have laws that ban discrimination based on sexual orientation, gender identity and gender expression. Many states recognize civil unions and an increasing number have legalized same-sex marriages. Public discussions related to sexual orientation, gender identity and gender expression are front and center. Hopefully the conversation is happening in your family as well.

Help your child understand that:

- Sexual orientation and gender identity are fundamental parts of who we are.

- No one can cause another person to be gay, lesbian or heterosexual.

- Having sexual thoughts and feelings about, or even experiences with, someone of the same gender does not necessary mean that a person is gay or lesbian.

• People of all sexual orientations and gender identities deserve healthy, loving relationships.

Encourage your children to ask questions and talk about their feelings. Ask them what they've heard from kids at school. This may bring up anxieties they're having about their own sexual development. In addition to reassuring them, let them know your own values and perspectives.

Be clear that it's wrong to discriminate against someone because of their sexual orientation, gender identity or gender expression. It's not OK to make comments like "that's so gay" — a phrase typically used to describe something that's stupid or foolish. It's not OK to laugh when someone else makes that statement. Point out words that are often used to be hurtful or to ridicule or bully another person.

Emphasize that people who are gay, lesbian and transgender have loving relationships, partnerships and marriages. And ultimately, be sure that your children know you love, accept and support them for who they are.

Tell me I'm OK

Young people can be pretty anxious and insecure about the many physical and emotional changes they experience during puberty. They worry about their bodies: *"Am I too short? Too tall?" "Why am I so flat chested?" "When will my penis grow?" "I hate my nose!" "When do I start growing and changing... all of my friends are." "What's wrong with me?"*

They feel awkward and uncoordinated as arms and legs grow completely out of sync with one another. Their moods are erratic for no apparent reason. Of course, it wouldn't be cool to ask anybody about this stuff… or worse yet, they may not think they have anyone in their lives they can trust enough to ask. So they often just fret in silence. Confidence and self-esteem can take a nosedive during puberty.

Self-esteem is something that parents have helped foster (or not) in their children since birth. From very early on, children have experiences that affect how they feel about themselves. For example: If mom's angry about the way Lucas is behaving, does she make it clear that she still loves *him* and that it's his behavior – not Lucas himself – that's not OK? When Lilly attempts a new skill, is she praised for *trying* – or only if she succeeds? When Gavin is worried that he's inferior to his peers, does his dad simply say, *"It's not a big deal,"* or does he remind Gavin that whatever his differences or limitations (whether physical, intellectual… whatever), these help to make him the unique and special person he is?

As parents, we can offer our children understanding, respect, applause and recognition. We can help them build confidence, and as we acknowledge their successes we can also teach them about learning from their mistakes, failures or challenges.

Along with this, we can ensure that our children have complete and accurate information about the physical, emotional and sexual changes that are all part of growing up. Having the facts makes the unknown less scary and less likely to cause the confusion and worry that so often rattle that sense of being OK in the world.

The **Middle School** Years

This too shall pass

You don't get it. You've always been rather proud of the talks you and your child had in the past about sexual issues. They seemed comfortable and straightforward. You've done your best to answer questions honestly, to initiate conversations, to affirm that sexuality is a wonderful and positive part of who we are.

So what happened? Suddenly your sixth-grader has decided the topic is off-limits. S/he's horrified (resistant/embarrassed/nervous — take your pick) whenever the subject comes up. Where did this go wrong?

Welcome to life with a middle schooler. This is a time when the topic of sexuality becomes much more personal and close to home… and you're much more likely to hear, *"I don't want to talk about this!"* We're at a whole other level now, when parents need to muster patience, understanding and creative thinking to keep those lines of communication with their children open. Here are a few tips:

- **Continue** bringing up the subject where it makes sense, but keep it light; don't push. Settle for a one-way discussion if need be… at least it's putting out your message. You might be surprised what your child retains, even when she doesn't seem to be listening.

• **Avoid** preaching. As the teen years approach, it's tempting for parents to fall into lecture mode. A litany of "do this... don't do that" can trigger kids to tune out or resist conversations with mom and dad even more. When parents truly listen to *their* children and are interested in their thoughts and opinions, it encourages communication.

• **Encourage** your child to think about and share his own ideas about sexual issues. Be prepared to hear that some of his views are different from yours. *Make it safe for him to question or disagree.* Let him know that your love and support don't depend on his agreement with your views.

• **Acknowledge** your child's reactions. Say something like, *"You look uncomfortable talking about this. Other than not talking about it at all, how can we make it easier?"*

• **Acknowledge** your own feelings... for example, *"I feel frustrated when I think you might be tuning me out. I'd like to be able to talk about this together."*

• **Invest** in some of the wonderful sexuality books written for young people. Leave them around the house.

• **Keep** your sense of humor... and use it generously.

This is actually a great time to talk about sex

In a 2011 national poll, 82% of parents with children ages 10 to 18 said they were talking with their kids about a range of sexuality topics including relationships, when it's OK to have sex, and their values about these issues. Fewer parents discussed birth control or how to say no to sex (Let's Talk: Are Parents Tackling Crucial Conversations about Sex?, Planned Parenthood Federation of America and the Center for Latino Adolescent and Family Health at the Silver School of Social Work at New York University). Most parents see the importance of sexuality education and want to be part of providing it. They want to help their children be healthy and safe. Many are also unprepared for the depth of information and skills that young people should be learning, even during the middle school years.

Some parents worry that talking about birth control and sexual protection sends a message that condones or even promotes having sex. Not so. Research has shown that young people who have open and factual discussions about sex with their parents are more likely to delay having sex. When they do become involved in a sexual relationship, they're more likely to protect themselves with condoms and/or birth control.

It takes some foundation work to build up to the fairly detailed conversations parents and their children need to have about these things. Don't wait to introduce the topics until your child is well into the teen years. For the majority of 12-year-olds, these more advanced sexual issues can still be addressed at a fairly non-threatening, non-emotional level, since most people this age are not yet personally involved. That's less likely to be the case a few years down the road. And once the issues become more pertinent in their lives, the discussions can be more challenging.

Boyfriends... girlfriends?

You're likely to have a few ideas about when your child will be old enough to have a boyfriend/girlfriend. Your child likely has ideas about that too – and they may be very different from yours. It's a common parent lament that kids are pressured to grow up too fast these days. Be that as it may, parents play an important role in helping their children develop relationships that are healthy, respectful and safe.

According to surveys conducted by The National Campaign to Prevent Teen and Unplanned Pregnancy, teens say that parents have the greatest influence on their decisions about relationships. Your children are watching you model how to treat others and how they themselves should expect to be treated in relationships. This is a great age to have conversations about what makes a good friend, girlfriend, boyfriend, partner. It's also a time to acknowledge how new, exciting and powerful these feelings and attractions can be. So it's important to be thoughtful about what you tell your children, and have clear expectations and boundaries in mind.

We don't want children to be pushed into social situations they're not ready for or old enough for. We also realize that even elementary school children play with the notion of boyfriends and girlfriends. As you become aware of this among your child's peer group, grab the opportunity to hear their thoughts about what those relationships are all about. Be a listener in this conversation before jumping in with what you think about things. Be sensitive to the fact that these interests and attractions may not all be toward people of the other gender.

Early activities with a "boyfriend" or "girlfriend" may include the usual scribbling of hearts or initials on notebooks, or passing or texting notes. Unfortunately, some sixth-graders (more often sixth grade girls with older boys) get involved in sexual experimenting... a sobering thought. It's not too early to talk about feelings and pressures that sometimes go along with interest in romantic relationships. This is another example of addressing an issue *before* (hopefully) it becomes a problem! You can help prepare your youngster for the fun, excitement and responsibility of such relationships, as well as the frustration, uncertainty and disappointment that sometimes results.

There are skills involved in developing positive, healthy relationships — skills that can be taught and fostered throughout childhood. But young people are less likely to look to their parents for guidance if they think they will be teased, not taken seriously, or met with, *"You're too young to have a boyfriend/girlfriend."*

The media... the message

The media landscape has been evolving at breakneck speed, and most young people are fully engaged in it. Cable and satellite dishes beam countless television shows into homes; the Internet serves up a banquet of web sites including social networking opportunities; cell phones, music and video games provide dozens of entertainment options. All of this adds up to considerable media time for youth. A 2010 study found that the average daily media usage for young people ages 8 to 18 includes TV and/or Internet movies ($4^{1}/_{2}$ hours), computer use outside of school work ($1^{1}/_{2}$ hours), music ($2^{1}/_{2}$ hours), and texting/talking on a cell phone ($1^{1}/_{2}$ hours) (Generation M2: Media in the Lives of 8- to 18-Year-Olds, Kaiser Family Foundation, January 2010).

How can parents set up reasonable guidelines and expectations that allow their children to take advantage of the benefits of media in ways that are smart, responsible and safe?

Talk with your children about their media use and that of their peers. Listen to what they like about popular music, TV shows, web sites, phone apps, and other media. Take some time to experience this media *with* your children, using that time to connect and share thoughts – or concerns – each of you might have about messages or values reflected in the media.

Use good judgment to monitor your children's media activities. Sometimes parents panic about keeping their children safe online and rush to install blocks or filters that also wind up preventing access to useful

Sometimes parents panic about keeping their children safe online and rush to install blocks or filters that also wind up preventing access to useful sources of information.

sources of information. That's not to say there isn't a place for filters, especially with younger children. However, they can't take the place of frank discussions with your children about the very issues you're looking to protect them from. Be careful not to have a false sense of security. Despite house rules and expectations, blocks and filters, children will encounter inappropriate media at some point. Your children's exposure to media – the good and the awful – gives you the chance to talk with them and help them develop filters through which they can sort, interpret and evaluate media messages. Empower them to be informed media consumers.

The web site www.pbs.org/parents/childrenandmedia offers tools for parents who are raising children – from preschool through high school – in the digital age. The site provides age-specific tips and discussion ideas about four media categories: TV and movies, computers, video games, and advertising. By being an active participant in your children's media use, you work with them to develop critical thinking skills that help them be more informed, aware and careful.

Reliable resources

Can you remember some of the crazy things you heard from your peers about sex when you were growing up? That might be something you can share with your own children as a way to start a conversation about reliable resources. *"When I was your age I heard that you couldn't get pregnant the first time you had sex. I also remember this idea that if you had sex, it meant you were a grown-up. I'm wondering if those myths are still out there today. What kinds of things do you hear people your age saying about sex?"*

Let your child know that when it comes to sexuality, it's important that he have accurate information and caring adults he can turn to who are reliable and honest with him. Encourage your child to think of you as one of those caring adults... and acknowledge that there may be times when, for whatever reason, he may choose not to come to you with questions or concerns. Ask if he can identify others he

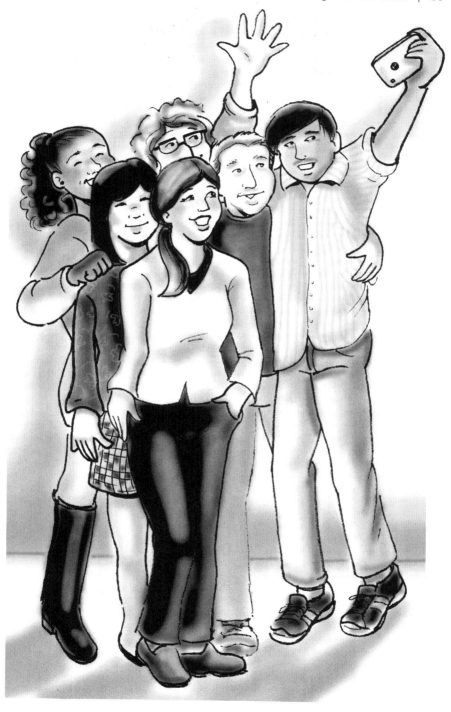

would feel comfortable turning to. Another parent? A teacher or school counselor? An aunt, uncle or other family member?

Also, mention that often when people have questions related to sexual issues, they simply Google them. There are many useful web sites available. There's also a lot of junk on the Internet, ranging from questionable to potentially dangerous. It's important to make sure the web site is reputable before accepting the answer (see Resource Section for useful sites).

If young people have several options for finding information, support and guidance on sexuality issues, they may feel a bit less inclined to accept their peers as the "sexperts."

How can you make it safer for your child to discuss sexuality with *you?*

- **Recognize** that many young people are wondering about a range of sexual issues that never occurred to you at that age. If you're tempted to think, *"He's a little young for this information, isn't he?"* remember the environment we live in.

- **Listen more than talk**. Hear his concerns and questions. Understand that his interest in the subject doesn't mean he or his friends are having sex or considering it.

- **Respect** that he may express views or ideas that differ from yours. Ask him to help you better understand why he thinks or feels the way he does.

- **Provide** factual information *and* let him know your values.

- **Trust** his ability to make good decisions when he has accurate information, good skills and your support.

Let your child know — by your words *and* your actions — that sex is a good topic to talk about in the family.

Puberty 101... refresher

Let's revisit puberty one more time. Puberty can start as early as age 8; it often begins at 10 or 11, but for some it is even later; and it's a fairly lengthy process, on average taking three to five years to complete. There's a good chance that during sixth to eighth grade, your child is in the thick of it. As with many topics, it deserves ongoing conversation. Hopefully you spent some time preparing your son or daughter for puberty back in fourth grade, but the issue is likely even more relevant now.

Puberty. Almost sounds like a disease. For those experiencing it, it can *feel* like one. Of course, much of that has to do with the incredible changes that are happening: hormones surging, bodies transforming (usually into sizes and shapes that never seem quite right), hair growing in places it hasn't before.

Then there's that emotional roller coaster that often accompanies puberty: intense feelings of excitement, attraction, anxiety, happiness, anger, dissatisfaction... perhaps all within a matter of hours! It's so important for kids to hear that, while seemingly weird and maddening, everything they're going through is pretty typical.

Even though they're dying for answers and reassurance, many young people have a hard time letting parents in on their concerns. Don't mistake their silence as a sign that they know it all or don't want to talk about it. Sometimes their confusion is so great, they're not even sure what to ask or how to begin. Add the awkwardness that often goes along with conversations about sexuality issues... and you can appreciate their dilemma.

If your memories of puberty have mellowed over time, here are some of the pressing concerns:

"I'm the tallest (shortest, skinniest, fattest) kid in the class. I hate it!"

"Will my penis ever grow?"

"Why am I so flat-chested?"

"I'm the only girl I know who hasn't gotten 'it' (my period). What's wrong with me?"

"What do I do with these new (sexual) feelings and thoughts I'm having (for people of the same or other sex)?"

"What do my friends think of me?"

"Am I normal???"

Spare your children some anxiety by talking about how this puberty business works. Tell them stories about your own experiences going through puberty and how you managed them. How old were you when it started? What did you notice? How did it feel? What were your worries? Where did you find support? Use humor. Use books – or leave them lying around the house (see Resource Section for suggestions). There are a number of helpful web sites designed to help young people decipher what's happening to them (for example, check out www.kidshealth.org/teen/sexual_health).

Remind your children that people grow and change at their own rate, whether they like it or not, and that they develop at the time that's right for them. Some start early, some late... either way, it's normal. Puberty generally takes several years to complete, and throughout that time there are a series of physical changes that follow a somewhat predictable order. Lots of young people follow a slightly different order – and that's normal too!

(Note: Some children have uncharacteristic anatomy and sex development that may have been identified at birth. For others, those differences may go undetected until puberty. Depending on the condition, these young people may go through puberty differently than others. There may be additional decisions for them to make, which will bring the need for additional information, support and reassurance. See Resource Section for books and web sites that can help.)

Remember to talk with your kids about more than just the physical changes. Emerging sexual feelings, emotions, relationships and stresses are all part of the journey, and can be especially difficult for them to identify — much less talk about. Let them know that even if they feel like they can't come to you, it's important they have other resources for accurate information, reassurance and support. Help them identify who and what those resources might be. Continue to be available, open and ready to talk. You just might be surprised when they take you up on the offer.

Reality check

"How do you make a baby?" Remember the first time your little one asked THE QUESTION? It really caught you off guard (maybe you just never expected the issue to crop up at such an early age).

That little one is now in seventh grade... perhaps with parents who are still caught off guard when it comes to sexuality and youth. Sexual involvement, unintended pregnancy, HIV and AIDS, sexually transmitted diseases (STDs, which are sometimes referred to as sexually transmitted infections), birth control and sexual protection... as parents, we don't expect these issues to become relevant at such an early age for *our* kids, right?

CONSIDER:

- According to the 2013 national Youth Risk Behavior Survey from the Centers for Disease Control and Prevention (CDC):

  - Nearly 47% of students (ninth through 12th grade) have had sexual intercourse.

  - 5.6% of students had sexual intercourse for the first time before age 13.

· Among youth who are currently sexually active, only 59.1% used a condom the last time they had sexual intercourse.

● Gay, lesbian and bisexual students are at greater risk of unhealthy sexual (and other) behaviors (Morbidity and Mortality Weekly Report, CDC, June 2011).

● Nearly half of all new cases of STDs occur in people between the ages of 15 and 24 (Sexually Transmitted Diseases Surveillance, CDC, 2010).

These young people are similar to the friends and schoolmates of your own children. They may *be* your own children, your nieces and nephews. They come from all socioeconomic levels, racial and ethnic groups, and religious affiliations. They reflect the need for sexuality education, for support in having healthy relationships, for access to services and support that help young people be healthy and safe. It's most effective when parents talk with their children about intercourse and other sexual activities, teenage pregnancy and STDs early on − *before* these issues become possibilities for them or their peers.

Most seventh-graders are capable of understanding the broader implications of sexual relationships. Not yet deeply involved themselves, they may be better able to have more casual, rational discussions with mom and dad about why some teens might choose to have sex, the responsibilities involved, and possible outcomes. It can work well to have a number of these chats while driving in the car... perhaps it's less intimidating than sitting down face-to-face.

In your conversations, remember to include the part about sex being for pleasure and not just to make babies. Parents can get caught up in their fears about teens having sex and default to only talking about the risks. This is another chance for parents to listen to what their children think about these things, clear up misinformation, and voice personal values and beliefs in a non-threatening, non-judgmental manner.

A little help from friends...

The depth of sexuality education important for a seventh-grader may be more than parents realize. You might be thinking, *"Are you kidding? I didn't know half of that stuff until I was out of college! A lot of it I'm still not sure about!"*

It's true. Today's young people are asked to manage some pretty sophisticated and complex issues. Parents often notice gaps in their own sexual knowledge when they try to offer information and guidance. It's easy to feel overwhelmed about what to say and how to begin. Really, it's not about being an expert. You'll learn specifics and practical "how to's" of sex education as you go along. And you can learn together *with* your children.

Think about your own resources. Perhaps you are part of a faith community with a youth pastor or faith leader who can be helpful. What about your family doctor, your child's pediatrician, or a family counselor? There's always Planned Parenthood and other local agencies that serve youth and families. And don't forget the Internet. There are many sites that are useful... here are just a few:

- www.plannedparenthood.org

- www.advocatesforyouth.org

- www.siecus.org

- www.hhs.gov/ash/oah

What about porn?

You can think of it as another teachable moment. It's very common for children to actively seek out or stumble upon pornographic web sites and magazines, so why not have some discussions in advance about that (which is so much easier than having to react in the moment)?

Even if you discover that your child has intentionally viewed pornography on occasion, please... don't freak out. Easy to say and tough to do, right? You might be really angry. Or anxious that something's wrong with your child. Or worried that viewing pornography is harmful. Still, an overreactive, angry or shaming response can be more damaging than pornographic images. *Really.*

Some pornography includes violence, but according to Marty Klein, a family and sex therapist, most of it doesn't because there's not a large market for that (Sexually Smarter: Your Kids Look at Porn. Now What?, January 2012). He encourages parents to be forthright and open in their discussions with their children... ideally *before* they discover the telltale search history on their child's computer or find the magazine or DVD under the bed.

Take time to think through how you want to play this. Remember some of the fundamentals: young people's interest in sex is normal; during adolescence, curiosity – as well as sexual thoughts, feelings and fantasies – are heightened, sometimes dramatically so. Think about why young people look at porn: curiosity, of course; because their friends do, and they want to fit in or be cool; for stimulation (yes, it can be difficult or uncomfortable to acknowledge that your child is a sexual being, *as are all humans, young and old).*

So what do you want him to know? First and foremost, that you love him. And you have some concerns that the two of you need to talk about. Young people need to hear that it's natural to be interested in sex and curious about bodies (especially – but not only – those of the gender they're sexually attracted to). However, it's important for him to know that pornographic images of sex do not represent real life or real relationships. The people involved are acting and are usually paid for their performances. As with other media, there's a lot of editing that goes on to make the images more appealing to consumers. There are camera shots that enhance sexual body parts, makeup, airbrushing... most people don't really look like that.

Encourage your child to ask questions about anything he has seen or is confused about. Tell him you understand that it probably feels uncomfortable or awkward to be having this conversation with you, and that parents and kids don't often talk with each other about sex (unfortunately). It's likely far fewer talk about pornography. Let him know that's not what *you* want. Even if it's challenging, you're going to help him get good information. You're going to let him know what you think about things, and you're going to listen to what he thinks.

Some parents put the computer in a shared family space, which limits their child's private access; others install filters or blocking software on the computer. There's certainly an age and a place for these kinds of measures. There are a number of tools and web sites that can help parents consider this decision in a thoughtful way (for example: www.safekids.com/child-safe-search). As our kids get older, it's important and appropriate for them to have more privacy, more independence. We want to respect that while preparing them to be smart, confident and safe.

Of course, the bottom line is that parents need to decide for themselves what path they want to take in handling this issue. Whatever that path is for you, remember that nothing can take the place of the clear, honest and loving conversations you have with your children, the information and values you share. These help create the most effective filters your children can carry with them, no matter where they are or what media they use.

When will I be ready?

"My friends talk a lot about getting girlfriends, but I'm just not interested in that. Am I weird or something?"

"I wish I was popular like Leila. All the boys like her."

Middle schools are filled with many who fret, *"What's wrong with me?!"*

Disappointment, bruised self-esteem, hurts and secret fears are rarely expressed to *anyone* – especially parents. Pressure to be involved in relationships increases their anxiety. And when young people are attracted to someone of their own gender, particularly in an unsupportive environment, it can feel even more isolating.

Reassure your child that people develop social readiness at their own rate. Acknowledge how confusing it can be to have friends who vary greatly on that readiness scale. Even if your child hasn't shown any concerns about this, bring it up... just to be sure. Break the ice with your own recollections of middle school:

"I remember there being lots of talk about boyfriends and girlfriends. Me? I could have cared less at the time, but I didn't dare admit it. My friends would have never let me live it down! But you know, some of them secretly felt the same way I did."

"I also wonder about young people who are attracted to people of their own gender. With all that pressure to have a boyfriend or girlfriend, I imagine they feel pretty cut off and afraid to talk about their feelings."

These kinds of comments can be nice conversation starters. At the very least, they let your children know that you're paying attention, you're interested, and you're there for them. It gives them permission to follow their own pace and acknowledges the many pressures that young people feel to move faster than they are ready for... all of which can lead to conversations about managing those pressures. It also opens the door should your children be questioning their own sexuality.

You just might be able to help relieve some of the social pressures your children are experiencing. Talk about feelings and situations that can arise when romantic interests and sexual attractions begin to grow. Even if your child isn't ready (or willing) to talk freely about this, you won't be wasting your time. The message will still be heard: *"If you're feeling confused about this, please know that I'm here for you. I'll listen, try to understand, and I might even be able to help."*

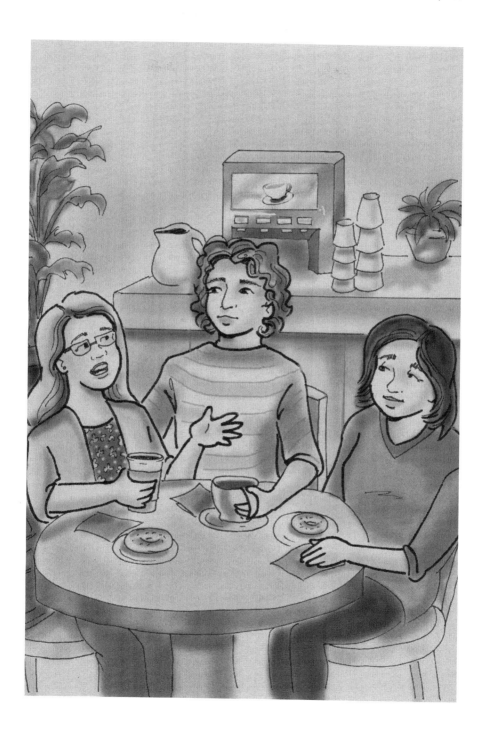

What do I say about...

When it comes to discussing sexual values with your children, *say what you believe.* It's that simple (or that difficult). Sex before marriage. Masturbation. Contraception. Teen pregnancy. Gay marriage. Gender issues. Pornography. When there's trust, safety and opportunity, young people ask lots of questions about these and other sexual topics. They want information... *and* they want to hear what you think.

Sometimes parents aren't quite sure *how* to have these discussions – or even whether it makes sense to talk about these issues at this age. They may opt to avoid the subject altogether unless their kids bring it up. That's a missed opportunity. It can give the impression that mom or dad would rather not talk about it. So by default, the only messages or values your children receive are those that come from others.

Sound familiar? – ***"I don't want to encourage her," or "I don't want my son to think that as long as teens use birth control, it's OK for them to have sex."***

This is a common worry, but information does not equal encouragement or permission. If you set out your value that sex is for marriage, or sex is for adults (or whatever you believe), and then talk with your child about the importance of birth control and sexual protection, are you giving a contradictory message? Young people can understand when parents give factual information while being clear about their values. For example: *"I believe teens should not have sex until they're older. I also realize that many do. It's important that people protect themselves from pregnancy and sexually transmitted diseases."*

With One Voice, a periodic survey conducted by The National Campaign to Prevent Teen and Unplanned Pregnancy, asked young people ages 12 to 19, "Suppose a parent or other adult tells a teen the following: *'I strongly encourage you to not have sex. However, if you do, you should use birth control or protection.'* Do you think this is a message that encourages teens to have sex?" Seventy-one percent said no. In that same survey, most young people stated that they wished young people were getting information about both abstinence and contraception rather than either/or.

Sound familiar? – ***"I don't want to preach."***

Excellent, because your children don't want that either. Be clear with them about *your* personal beliefs… and ask about *theirs* and those of their peers. It's a conversation, not a sermon. For example, a parent might say, *"I believe teens are too young to have sex. I'm not sure they're prepared for the emotions and responsibilities that go along with a sexual relationship. There are good reasons to wait. What is your sense about that?"* or *"I'm guessing young people might be feeling pressure to have sex before they feel ready. That was true in my day, and I assume it's even more so now. Am I right about that? What do young people do when they experience that pressure? I wouldn't want them to regret their decision."*

You might also say, *"My hope is that you know you can come to me if you're ever wrestling with decisions about sex. I'll do all I can to listen and offer you information and guidance you can consider in making your choice. My highest priority is your well-being, so I want you to be informed."*

A genuine give-and-take of ideas can allow your child to sort out the issues and draw some conclusions, hopefully before s/he is confronted with making the choices.

Ultimately our children form their own opinions and develop their own values, which may or may not be in line with ours. You might be surprised by how much alignment there is at the end of the day, though. As they develop and go through the process of discovering who they are and what they value, young people need to examine, question, challenge. Would you rather your child test out ideas and views about sexuality in an arena of open communication with you – or through experimentation?

Oh right... that values piece

Even parents who were fairly open and upfront about sexual discussions when their children were little often find themselves struggling once the adolescent years hit.

The issues are far more complex... and it's more than that. Parent-child roles change significantly as kids get older. With small children, parents essentially set the rules, promote the values, and select the paths for learning and growth. With adolescents, parents discuss (perhaps negotiate) rules and offer a rationale for their importance. Values continue to be emphasized and promoted... but at times with a panicked assertiveness (which can trigger anger, frustration... and an end to the conversation). Parents often have a very real fear that their children may balk at some core beliefs and attitudes they want them to embrace.

Ultimately, teens challenge and test their parents' values, then accept, modify or reject them. A number of studies show that adolescents do adopt many of the family's basic values, even more so when parents provide structure in a nurturing, democratic (rather than a controlling or authoritarian) way.

You can create a safe environment within the family for your children to discuss or question differing values. Encourage them to think out loud, to examine beliefs and the possible impact of going with (or against) them. Frank discussions in which parents and children listen to and speak with (not at) one another enhance young people's ability to make thoughtful choices.

Confusing connections?

"I understand this business of same-gender role models and confidants during adolescence. What I don't understand is this intense 'attachment' Gabel has to his teacher, Mr. Brown. It's as though Gabel has a crush on the guy! Is this... normal?"

It's not necessarily an indication that Gabel is gay, if that's what you mean. It's common for adolescents to develop a strong connection to a same-gender person of importance in their lives: a teacher, coach, perhaps even a classmate. This person might be someone they greatly admire or someone they want to be like. The special bond they have with this person often allows them to feel safe, to seek advice, or to share their feelings and concerns. They may try to spend as much time as possible with this person, and may even feel jealous or upset if the relationship changes.

Such feelings can be terribly confusing to a young person and to parents.

Teens often have confusion, questions and anxieties about relationships and sexual issues in general, including sexual orientation. *"How can you tell if a person's gay?" "If someone masturbates, does that mean s/he's gay?" "Lisa and Ann are always together. They must be more than just friends, don't you think?"*

Some people know as young children that they're gay; others become clear about this in their teens, or even later. While the acronym has changed over time, the Q in LGBTQ* sometimes stands for Questioning... and young people can be very much in this stage of questioning their sexuality.

Regardless of whether your children are straight or gay, if you're concerned about any of their relationships or suspect they may have concerns, talk with them about it. Have conversations about what makes a healthy friendship, including the importance of honesty and respect in a relationship — no hidden motives or manipulation. In a healthy relationship, people care about each other with no strings attached. If that's not the case, maybe it's time to reconsider the relationship.

* Lesbian, Gay, Bisexual, Transgender, Questioning. Q can also stand for "Queer," a reclaimed word of pride for some.

More about relationships

It's never too soon to talk with your children about unhealthy relationships or dating violence. Conversations should start even before they begin dating. Data from the 2013 Youth Risk Behavior Survey showed that nationwide, among the nearly 74% of high school students who had dated within the previous 12 months, 10.3% had been intentionally hit, slapped or physically hurt by the person they were dating. Lesbian, gay, bisexual and transgender youth are at higher risk of dating violence, according to a 2013 report from the Urban Institute. Abusive and violent relationships can begin early for young people and last throughout their lives.

Intimate partner violence takes many forms, not just physical. There is also emotional abuse, such as name calling, belittling, bullying, or keeping a partner away from friends and family; electronic violence, including constant texting or posting sexual pictures of a partner on social media pages; and sexual violence, such as coercing or forcing a partner to take part in a sexual behavior when s/he does not want or is not in a condition to consent to. There is reproductive coercion, which can include being dishonest about contraceptive use or interfering with a partner's contraception, all in an effort to gain power and control.

> *Everyone deserves to have healthy and safe relationships (romantic and otherwise). Help your children recognize what these types of relationships look and feel like. One of the best ways to do this is to demonstrate healthy relationships with your partner or spouse, friends, and your own children.*

Everyone deserves to have healthy and safe relationships (romantic and otherwise). Help your children recognize what these types of relationships look and feel like. One of the best ways to do this is to demonstrate healthy relationships with your partner or spouse, friends, and your own children.

Talk with your kids about what they look for in a friend, boyfriend or girlfriend. Help them be concrete in their descriptions. For instance, if they say, *"Someone who's nice," "Someone who respects me," "Someone who's supportive,"* ask for examples of what each of those qualities might look and feel like. What are some things a person does that show s/he is being nice, respectful, supportive?

As young people begin to pay attention to what relationships are all about, they can begin to identify red flags of unhealthy or potentially abusive or violent relationships. Sometimes in the early stages of abusive relationships, the signs may not be as obvious or seem like that big of a deal. The power and control may build over time to the point where the person feels helpless or unable to get out.

Talk with your children about some of the warning signs... a friend or partner who:

- Constantly puts his/her needs in front of yours.

- Does not control his/her temper and acts out in anger.

- Is possessive — tries to keep you away from your friends and family.

- Tells you how to dress, where to go or what to do.

- Checks your cell phone without asking.

- Constantly tracks your online friends.

- Puts you down.

- Is extremely jealous.

- Threatens to hurt him/herself – or you – if you end the relationship.

No one deserves to be abused. If your children find themselves in that kind of relationship, they need to hear that the abuse is not their fault. They need to know they shouldn't feel embarrassed or ashamed. Urge your children: If they or someone they know is in an unhealthy, abusive or violent relationship, they should immediately tell someone who can help... a parent, teacher or other trusted adult.

There are several online resources designed specifically for youth who are, or worry that they might be, in an unhealthy relationship. Check out www.loveisrespect.org or a similar site listed in the Resource Section.

Intentional parenting

The Search Institute, an organization whose mission is "To create a world where all young people are valued and thrive" (www.search-institute.org), has identified 21 family assets that support positive outcomes for youth. One grouping of these assets relates to setting and maintaining expectations for children, including clear boundaries and fair rules.

Parental influence in the lives of children is powerful and important. Work together with your teens to establish clear expectations for behavior, curfews and rules, as well as the appropriate consequences if rules are broken. Follow through (that's often the hardest part, right?).

Know who your children's friends are, and get to know their parents. Ask your children where they are going, who they will be with and when they will be home. Unsupervised time at home is one contributing factor to teen sexual activity and other behaviors that potentially put young people's health and safety at risk. If your teen wants to hang out at a friend's home, find out whether a parent or other adult will be there.

Monitor your children's Internet use, and be aware of what they're listening to, watching and reading. Have conversations with your children and help them think critically about the media they and their friends are using.

Be in communication, even when you're not together. Check in with teens, and be sure they always know how to get in touch with you. Build a safety plan with them in the event they find themselves in a situation that makes them feel like they may be in over their heads.

Effectively monitoring our children is best accomplished when there's a history of good communication, listening, mutual respect and consistency. Of course, this all sounds like good common sense and responsible parenting. It's the implementation that can get challenging. Young people can be masters of protest, foot stomping, eye rolling, door slamming and accusations of, *"You just don't trust me!"* Remind them that this isn't about not trusting them. It's about caring for their health and safety. It's about good parenting.

Media mania: sex sells

Parents recognize that while they strongly influence their children's lives, they're not the only ones. Young people hear and consider many voices: parents, friends, the media, health professionals, the clergy — each contributing influence and pressure, which can affect the decisions they make.

You can't guarantee that your kids won't have sex during their teen years. You can, however, make sure they have information, guidance and strategies in place to help them with the pressures that encourage sex among youth. The pressures are many and powerful, with some of the most potent and explicit coming from the media. Sex is used to sell everything from swimwear to burgers. Sitcoms and reality shows sizzle with sex. The Internet has opened up a world of ready access to sexual images from tame to porn.

The media affects people in many ways. The parade of "perfect" faces and figures can leave us feeling inadequate about our own bodies. For adolescents in a time of dramatic and usually awkward development, the impact can be especially hard. By suggesting that the ultimate love life and a hot body are of utmost importance, the media fosters unrealistic expectations. This can set teens up for disappointment and dissatisfaction with themselves and their relationships.

Sometimes the message is more subtle. Consider gender role expectations and stereotypes. Even in today's ads, for example, who's usually the spokesperson for laundry soap, diet foods, or quick and easy dinner menus? Women. According to research from Children Now (www.childrennow.org), nearly 40% of the female characters in video games are dressed in revealing clothes. When portraying females in positions of power, the media often shows women who are cold-hearted, angry or seriously challenged in relationships. Gender stereotyping is still alive and well in the media.

Male roles tend to be equally stifling. True, men are often cast as more assertive, independent, powerful, successful, intelligent... all characteristics that are viewed favorably. Yet they also model a lack of sensitivity, a one-track mind approach to relationships, and the "macho" image that discourages healthy social/emotional development in males.

The sadness of it all is that we've become so accustomed to such stereotypes in the media that we're almost oblivious to them!

We can empower young people by helping them be more alert to sexual messages and stereotypes of all kinds in the media. As a family, talk about how distortions in the media can influence attitudes and decisions connected to many sexual issues: body image, relationships, gender roles and expectations, readiness for sex and sexual responsibility.

The **High School** Years

What I really want to know is...

Young people aren't just curious about sex. They want to know about the whole business of living. They want to understand themselves and connect with others. How much does your teen know about you... or you about them?

Here's an exercise used in a parent-teen workshop offered by Planned Parenthood of Southwestern Oregon that opened up conversation about understanding, about connecting – and in some cases – about sex. It was structured like a mutual interview. If it's useful for you, you can adapt some of these discussion starters to use in more informal ways with your own children.

The starting point was making the following agreements:

1. What we talk about with each other is confidential.

2. We can be honest and not worry about judgment or consequences.

3. We can "pass" on any question.

The teens asked their parents:

- *What did you like most about being my age? What was really hard for you?*

- *What do you like best about being a parent? What's the hardest part?*

- *Tell me how I became part of our family, or, Tell me about the day I was born.*

- *What were your friends like when you were my age? Did you have a boyfriend or girlfriend? When were you allowed to go out... or whatever you called it back then?*

- *What was expected of you because of your gender? How did you feel about that? How do you feel about those expectations now?*

- *How do you feel about getting older?*

- *If you could change one thing about your body, what would it be?*

- *Did you ever make a really bad mistake when you were a teen? What did your parent(s) do?*

The parents asked their teens:

- *What do you like best about being your age? What's really hard for you?*

- *What would the best day of your life look like?*

- *What do you like about being your gender? What do you see as some of the difficult or negative things about being your gender?*

- *How do you decide who to be friends with?*

- *What do you wish we could talk about more openly?*

- *If you could travel ten years into the future, what do you suppose your life would look like?*

- *How do you feel about getting older?*

- *If you could change one thing about your body, what would it be?*

- *If you ever made a really bad mistake, is there an adult you could trust to talk with about it?*

Think about if and how you could have these kinds of discussions over time with your own children. These open-ended questions can help parents and teens gain insight into themselves and each other. And they have the potential of opening doors to meaningful conversations about love, sex and relationships.

Straining and gaining

Helping children make their way through adolescence can feel like an incredible challenge. Despite the wisdom gained from their own life experiences, parents often feel unprepared to advise teens on the issues they currently face. Some of the lessons from our own adolescence may not hold true for today's youth. It's tempting to equate adolescence with horror... but to the extent that parents focus on the difficulties and pain, they miss the joys.

Young people have two major tasks at hand:

1. Establishing independence — asserting themselves as separate and distinct from their parents.

2. Defining/clarifying their personal values.

Simultaneously, parents face their own tasks:

1. Letting go — allowing children the freedom to develop their separate identities.

2. Maintaining a climate of trust, safety and acceptance in which attitudes and values can be talked about, tested or challenged.

For parents, it's unsettling to accept that, *"I don't have the ultimate power to determine how my child's life will be."* Long before our kids become teens we recognize that, in the long run, they make their own decisions. But it's hard to give into that reality when the time comes.

Most parents are working hard to raise children to be responsible adults capable of making healthy (we hope) choices in their lives. Still, your teen may choose a path or adopt values that are different from your own or not what you'd prefer. That's difficult for parents to accept, particularly when some of the issues are *so very big:* relationships, sex, drugs.

As part of all this, parents are expected to let go and still provide guidance. What might that look like?

- **Giving** your children chances to make their own mistakes... then helping them learn lessons from those experiences.

- **Continuing** to speak about your values and beliefs... then accepting that your children may not fully embrace them.

- **Listening** without judgment (ooh, that's a tough one) to your children's views and opinions about things... and offering your input without insisting they are wrong.

The following is taken from Talking Back, a nationwide survey of teens conducted by The National Campaign to Prevent Teen and Unplanned Pregnancy. Here are some of the things young people said they wanted adults to know:

"Talk to us honestly about sex, love, and relationships. Just because we're young, doesn't mean that we can't fall in love or be deeply interested in sex."

"Telling us not to have sex is not enough. Explain why you feel that way, and ask us what we think."

"Whether we're having sex or not, we need to be prepared."

"Show us what good, responsible relationships look like. We're as influenced by what you do as by what you say."

"We hate 'The Talk' as much as you do. Instead, start talking to us about sex and responsibility when we're young, and keep the conversation going as we grow older."

You do your best... and there are no guarantees. Still, you can build the odds in your children's favor. Speak honestly with them about the power and excitement of attraction, being open to the possibility that they may feel attracted to the other sex, the same sex, both or neither. Talk with them about relationships and sex, about love and caring. Make sure they have the facts and insights they need to be prepared, informed and safe once they start having sex. Think about what you hope for your children, and let that help guide your message.

At this age, your children need to understand the range of sexual behaviors (not just vaginal intercourse!), possible risks associated with sexual behaviors, *and* ways to reduce those risks. They need practical information and the skills to make sexual decisions. Even if they are not making those decisions now, at some time, maybe in the not too distant future, they will be. Be clear about how pregnancy happens, how they can prevent sexually transmitted diseases, and where they can access contraception and sexual protection. *Underscore the importance of consent* — any sexual behavior that happens between people should be wanted and agreed to by each person. It's not just about saying no but about saying a clear yes. Don't assume they're getting any of this information in health class!

Continue to let your kids know your beliefs and values around these issues. Tell them that you hope they will wait to have sex until (they're older? out of high school? married? in a loving relationship?). You fill in the blank... just know it's important that they hear what you think – and *why*. Make sure they hear you say something like, *"Obviously I won't be there when you decide to have sex, so let me say this now, and hopefully you will remember: Your health and safety and your partner's health and safety are important. Protect yourselves."*

Many young teens do experiment with sexual behaviors – sometimes risky ones. It simply isn't enough for parents to say, *"Don't!"*

Peer power

Young people in relationships – both males and females – report feeling pressure to go further with sexual behaviors than they feel ready for. Sometimes that pressure comes from the mistaken notion that most of their peer group is having sex. And of course, for many young people there's a strong desire to fit in and be part of the group. But across the country, 53% of youth in grades nine to 12 have *not* had sex (Youth Risk Behavior Survey, Centers for Disease Control and Prevention, 2013). That's a good thing to tell your teen.

Parents feel anxious about peer pressure and social influences on their children's decisions. They worry that their own influence doesn't carry the same weight that it used to. With all good intent, some parents resort to just laying down the law: *"I don't want any argument... just do as I tell you."* That approach might get you what you're looking for in the short term. But as a long-term strategy it's not particularly helpful, and it can ultimately result in your child being resentful or even lying or sneaking around behind your back. Plus, you're losing the chance to help your teen see the bigger picture, learn about making thoughtful decisions, and figure out how to handle situations, challenges and pressures when you're not there.

Self-confidence, clear convictions and personal standards go a long way in helping young people avoid making choices based on outside pressures. It's important that parents set clear expectations and check in regularly with their teens to see how they're managing those expectations. When you monitor your children's activities, friends and whereabouts, it makes it less likely that they will engage in all kinds of risky behaviors, including having sex before they're ready.

Sometimes in the moment, a young person simply needs words to say or actions to take in a high-pressure situation. Help your teens think about ready responses to common pressure lines like, *"Why don't you want to have sex? I thought you cared about me."* Or, *"There's nothing to worry about. I'm on birth control."* Or, *"It's not such a big deal… most of our friends have already had sex."*

Make a game out of it — who can come up with the best response? Your conversation can be silly and fun… in fact, that can be helpful in breaking the ice. But ultimately, land on words and actions that your child can imagine feeling comfortable using in a high-pressure situation.

Acknowledge that you get how intense sexual feelings are, and that these normal, healthy feelings can be thrilling, scary and confusing — all at the same time. It can be tough to know how to handle them, especially if you're with someone you're really attracted to.

We can't just assume — no matter how many discussions we've had with them — that our children will feel confident about avoiding pressure situations. And sometimes situations arise that are unavoidable or beyond their control. Work with them on an exit plan. You might make an agreement that if your child winds up in a situation they're uncomfortable with and not sure how to handle, they can text or call you, and you will pick them up — no questions asked. You and your child can figure out the details of how to make that safety plan work. But talk about it now and have it in place in the event there's ever a need for it.

Help your children sort out the possible outcomes of their sexual decisions *before* they face the choices. Ask them to weigh the possible results of saying no to a sexual behavior, as well as saying yes. Talk about situations that can make it harder to say no to powerful sexual feelings... using alcohol or drugs, or spending time alone with someone rather than being together in a group. Talk with your teen about sharing love, affection and sexual feelings in ways that are responsible and appropriate at this age. Ask them what behaviors they think *are* responsible and appropriate, and let them know what *you* think.

Ultimately your teens are the ones to decide whether and when they will have sex, who they will have sex with, and what sexual behaviors they'll take part in. Let them know you expect them to be smart and caring in making those choices.

Full disclosure

As parents worry about teens having sex, it can be easy to focus on the dangers and not share the rest of the story. Talking with young people about intimacy and pleasure is just as important as making sure they understand any risks associated with sexual activities.

You should talk with your teen about sexual expression within the context of your own beliefs and values. Whether you wish to stress marriage, a mature and committed relationship, a particular age *("not while you're in high school")*, or some other indicator of readiness... please reinforce that sex, at the right time and with the right partner, can be amazing and wonderful. Yes, sexual relationships can also lead to problems, especially for the young, the uninformed, and the unprepared. But if we talk only about the negative side of sex, we're not being completely honest.

Are you concerned that it's not a good idea to talk with teens about sex being pleasurable, or that it might encourage them to try it? Newsflash: Teens already get that sex can feel really, really good. Usually, the only ones not talking with them about the joys and pleasures of sex are their parents. So you might want to bring that piece into the picture while you're helping them see the bigger context. And give your children credit: Talking about the obvious doesn't encourage them to go out and have sex. It might even open the door to deeper, more meaningful discussion.

Remember to be inclusive as you have these conversations. Your child might not be attracted to someone of another gender. Leave space for that and choose your language accordingly. It's important for young people to understand that "having sex" means different things to different people. We can't assume that it's male with female or that it's vaginal intercourse; we can't assume that "using protection" refers only to birth control and/or condoms; we can't assume that having sex implies the same level of connection, caring or commitment for each person. There are lots of assumptions about having sex that we can't or shouldn't make… whether it's parents talking with their teens about sex, or people thinking about having sex with each other.

Misunderstanding a partner's thoughts or expectations of what sex is all about can be hurtful. The experience can be disappointing at the very least, or filled with anxiety, guilt or regret. That's not what we want for our young people *whenever* sex becomes a part of their relationship. Let your teen know that once again, clear and honest communication is a key (and reoccurring) theme when it comes to having a healthy, positive and pleasurable sexual experience.

Talking with teens

"I've never really talked much with my daughter about sex. She's in 10th grade now… I suppose it's a little late, don't you think? Anyway, I guess she's learning what she needs to know in her health classes at school."

It's never too late to talk with your child about sex. OK… so ideally, these conversations start when children are small. If that hasn't happened, now's a good time to start. These discussions are important *throughout* your child's growing up years. And you may not want to be too quick to assume that your child's school is providing a comprehensive sex education curriculum. In fact, call the health teacher, school principal or director of instruction to find out just what is being covered. It's a chance for you to advocate for a comprehensive, research-based sex education program at school. Even if that is what's being provided in the classroom, *you're* the one who's in the best position to reinforce what's being taught *and* share values and expectations with your child.

Young people need more than just facts about sex. They want answers about the intangibles of sex. They're curious about the emotions, values and ethics involved in sexual relationships; they're both confused and excited about sexual feelings and urges; they wonder about love and how someone knows when they're ready for sex. Much of what they'd really like to know is highly personal... not health class material.

Surveys show that teens wish they could talk with their parents. So what gets in the way?

- *"I'm gay, and I just can't bring myself to tell my dad. I'm scared about how he'll take it."*

- *"If I ask my dad anything about sex, he'll think I'm having sex. And I'm not. . . I just wonder about a lot of things."*

- *"I'm still trying to figure out my own ideas about sex... like how do you know if it's the right time or the right person? My parents have pretty set ideas: you have sex when you're married. Period. I don't agree with that, but I can't talk to them about it. They would freak out."*

- *"My mom is still trying to understand that I'm transgender. Honestly, it makes it hard to talk with her about a lot of things."*

Sometimes teens avoid the subject because they think parents won't take them seriously:

- *"They still treat me like I'm a little kid. I can tell they think I don't need to know this stuff now."*

- *"If I even hint that I think some guy at school is cute, mom teases me. I doubt I could have a serious discussion with her about sex."*

Could similar concerns be getting in the way for your teen? A parent may not even suspect that their child feels this way. Think about initiating a conversation rather than waiting for your son or daughter to ask or bring up issues. Can you imagine, for example, sitting down with your son or daughter and saying something like:

"I really do care what you think about things. I know we won't always agree. That doesn't mean our relationship will fall apart. I will always love you, no matter what. I hope you feel you can come to me about anything: sex, drugs, relationships, school, whatever. I'll do my best to listen, understand and support you however I can. I don't often talk with you about these sorts of things because honestly… sometimes I feel a little awkward. And I don't want you to think I'm grilling you. But I want you to know that I am interested, and I'm here if you need me."

No matter what your child's age, it's never too late to open doors. You may have very different opinions about some very important issues. Can you accept that, and still keep the door open? Seen through adult eyes of experience, your teenager's concerns might at times seem trivial to you. Can you accept that, and still treat those concerns thoughtfully? While your child wants and needs your input, in the end s/he has to take charge and be allowed to grow and make personal decisions. Can you accept that, knowing that in the process s/he may choose differently than you hope, and that s/he will likely make mistakes?

It takes effort to build and maintain good communication habits — extra effort if parents and kids have not talked about these personal issues much in the past. Try now.

In his wisdom, the late Dr. Sol Gordon, an expert in the field of sexuality education, insisted that, "The quality of love and caring by parents or other important adults in a child's life is the single most significant component of a child's sex education.

What's a parent to do?!

This parenting business is an awesome task. We struggle to find the right answers, give appropriate guidance, and then sit back and hope for the best. And as parents are trying to manage the awesomeness of parenthood, their kids face the awesomeness of "kid-hood," which comes with its own intensity.

For a young person, one of the most important parts of growing up is gaining the necessary tools to make informed, responsible decisions about relationships and sex. Here are a few ways you might help in the process:

- **Be a healthy, positive role model.** Teens learn about love and intimacy by watching their parents and other adults relate to one another. You teach your children how to develop mature, loving relationships and how to cope with difficult ones through your behavior.

Help them see that sex is wonderful AND has its place as part of the larger picture. Emphasize respect, caring and communication as some of the critical pieces. In his wisdom, the late Dr. Sol Gordon, an expert in the field of sexuality education, insisted that, *"The quality of love and caring by parents or other important adults in a child's life is the single most significant component of a child's sex education."*

- **Stay connected.** Parents' expressions of love, attention and support are vital throughout your children's lives. While they may not ask for signs of affection from parents – and may even resist their parents' touch at times – teenagers need to feel and hear that they are loved. A hug or kiss, a squeeze of the hand, a pat on the back – whatever is comfortable and agreed upon – helps you stay "in touch" with your teen. Tell your child that you love them every day.

- **Promote a sense of the future.** Help your teen set and reach goals. Encourage their dreams and ambitions. Support them in considering educational and career options. Having a vision and goals for a bright future contribute to responsible choices.

- **Pay attention to the process.** Growing up is just that – a process. Chances to learn and gain insight occur all along the way. They're easily missed if adolescence is viewed as a race or survival course in which the sole purpose is getting to the end.

- **Talk with other parents.** Find out how other parents you know, respect and trust are helping their children be smart and thoughtful about relationships and sex. You may discover new or interesting approaches that had not occurred to you before.

The value of values

There's all this talk of sharing family "values" about sexuality… respecting that the values of others may be different from our own… the importance of acting on one's personal values.

Just what are these things called values anyway? Where do they come from? Do they change over time, and if so, does that mean they weren't really values in the first place?

Values are core beliefs that guide how we live. We may not recall consciously choosing our values. They just seem to be there, influencing our attitudes and behaviors. We can have difficulty explaining them to children. Parents may have little experience defining or examining their own values around sexuality and simply pass them on without much active discussion.

It's useful to revisit our core beliefs from time to time, to clarify and reaffirm what is true for us. This can be scary, since it forces us to examine what we say we value and what we truly value. It also forces us to take a good look at how well our behaviors match our stated beliefs. This "e-*value*-ation" can help us better guide our children in shaping their own personal values about sexuality.

The process of examining long-accepted ethics and standards of behavior is healthy, although it can also be painful. Parents confront the possibility that their children's values may not always line up with their own. And it's wonderful when they discover the common ground.

We teach children our values about sexuality through words and, perhaps more importantly, by modeling behaviors we see as right and just. The media and peers also promote certain values through the messages they deliver.

As they develop more independence, teens need to question, examine and test values. Then they can freely and consciously form their personal values, own their values, and build the conviction to live by them.

It's a difficult balance for parents: Striving to support their children in determining their own values while at the same time giving input and guidance. It requires trusting that young people are capable of choosing values that make sense for them in their lives. We can help our teens consider their values as we talk with them about issues like relationships, love, sex, gender identity, gender roles and expectations, sexual protection, contraception, sexual orientation, abortion, pregnancy, parenting, sexually transmitted diseases and more. Parents *and* teens need the freedom to express to one another what they know, feel, value and expect around each of these issues.

The following exercise can help clarify some values related to sexuality. Parents can do it alone and/or with their teens. For each statement, think (and talk) about why you agree, feel neutral, or disagree:

- *Sex outside of marriage is wrong.*

- *Teens should be able to get sexual protection and contraception without a parent's consent.*

- *Abortion should be legal.*

- *If a 15-year-old becomes pregnant, she should place the baby for adoption.*

- *Laws should support marriage equality whether it's a same-sex or different-sex couple.*

- *Gay and lesbian couples should have the freedom to adopt children.*

- *If a young person experiences a pregnancy as a teen, his/her parent(s) should help take responsibility for the baby.*

Your teen's relationships and sexual decisions will be affected by their ability to clarify, express, affirm and act on personal values. These are skills that improve with practice.

The art of setting limits

Young people need and want limits. Sure, they grumble, complain and generally storm around the house claiming, *"That's not fair! You're treating me like a baby! None of the other kids my age have these kinds of rules."* To which a typical (ineffective) parent response is often, *"I don't care about other kids. I care about you!"*

Sound familiar? It could be a replay from your own teen years. Remember the lines you swore you'd never use if you became a parent? Like: *"As long as you live in this house, you will live by my rules." "It doesn't matter that all the other kids stay out late. You're not the other kids." "I don't have to give you a reason. I said no. That's all there is to it!"*

Groan. More and more you hear yourself saying those very words you found so frustrating when you were a teen. You're not trying to be unreasonable. It's just that you're a parent now, with years of life experience, 20-20 hindsight, and your own memories of being in 10th grade. You want to protect your child. And if you're totally honest, you might admit that you worry about losing whatever control you may think you have left over this young adult. You know all about teens having sex, unplanned pregnancies, sexually transmitted diseases, HIV and AIDS. You feel somewhat justified retreating to the tactics your own folks used with you – the absolute restrictions meant for your own good.

Yet you know this approach can backfire. Unbending rules with no room to negotiate – or at least some conversation about the reasoning behind the rules – can cause resistance or rebellion in teens. Parents can't realistically lock them up. Sure, you can try to keep them from experimenting with sex by refusing to allow dating or by insisting on constant supervision. But you have to ask yourself, is that reasonable or even practical? And what are they learning in the process? How does that help them gain the skills they need to make their own smart, informed choices when adults are not around?

You can't and won't always be there. A big part of our job as parents is to help our children learn to think and act on their own… and then let them. They need to grow up and make decisions. A part of their job as teens is to take some risks. It gives them opportunities to try out their skills, explore their options, and find out who they are and what's important to them.

That doesn't mean they get to do whatever they want. It does mean that you work together to set limits. And yes, there is room for bottom-line requirements that are not negotiable… for example, *"Do not get in a car with someone who has been drinking. Text or call me, and I will pick you up, no questions asked."* Be upfront about your concerns and the basis for your decisions. It's neither sufficient nor effective to simply say, *"Because I'm your parent, that's why!"* That kind of statement closes the door to conversation and sets the stage for resentment. Instead, you might try this: *"I know sexual urges and feelings can be wonderful and so powerful. It's important we agree on some limits that help you stay in control of your decisions."*

Wherever you can, negotiate with your children to develop rules that are reasonable and that you can both live with. That process can help them learn about making decisions to manage their own behaviors. Work with your 10th-grader to set reasonable guidelines for afterschool free time and socializing with friends. Decide on specific afterschool routines and activities… homework, chores, organized programs, sports, etc. You can insist that friends not be in the house without an adult… at which your child will probably squawk, *"I can't believe this! Don't you trust me?"* And you might say, *"This isn't about trust. It's about helping you avoid difficult situations that you may have trouble handling."*

Make agreements that reduce the potential for problems: Parties must be chaperoned by a parent or responsible adult, no alcohol or drugs, and dating only in groups for now. Be clear about the consequences of not keeping the agreement… and follow through. Set up a reasonable curfew and a means of checking in if a situation feels uncomfortable or things are getting out of hand. When your kids have a clear sense of your expectations *and* understand the reasoning behind them, and when they have a part in helping make the rules, they're more likely to follow them – and they learn from the process.

Parents want to minimize the chances of kids getting into situations they're not ready to handle. Young people want to avoid that too. Yet they may not have developed skills to anticipate or manage those situations. So they're relieved to have the limits, and grateful to use mom or dad as an excuse when they need one. Of course, they won't admit that they appreciate the boundaries, but that's also part of being a teenager… remember?

Let's talk sexting

Experts differ on just how many young people are involved in sexting – sending sexually explicit pictures or messages through their cell phones. It's yet another one of those topics that parents panic about – especially since every few months or so, the media comes out with yet another story about the supposed "epidemic" of teen sexting. There have been high profile sexting cases where teens were prosecuted for dealing in child pornography and labeled sex offenders. In one tragic case, a young woman in Ohio committed suicide after a nude photo she had sent her boyfriend was circulated around her high school.

It's important to have forthright discussions with your teens about sexting, just as you would for any sexual health issue. And as with any sexual health issue, it's important to put it in perspective.

In today's world, teens are pretty comfortable – unfortunately too comfortable at times – sharing their lives online. Along with texting, Instagram, Snapchat, Whisper, Facebook and other social media sites and mobile apps have become part of young people's daily routine. Posting photos, instant messaging, connecting with friends and family… the technology has a lot of upsides and downsides. Technology is second nature for young people. It's the way they communicate and it's what they use to relate with one another. Because they can sometimes be impulsive at this age, some teens will send messages or photos without taking time to think through what they're doing.

From a young person's perspective, sexting can be seen as a fun and flirty thing to do. They don't realize the potential consequences of their actions. Help them think it through. There are a number of web sites that offer parents good insights and suggestions for talking with their children about safe and smart technology use. Here are just a few:

- www.commonsensemedia.org

- www.advocatesforyouth.org

- www.connectsafely.org

- www.thenationalcampaign.org/sextech

The basic tips include:

- **Ask questions.** Find out what your teens think about sexting. Have they or someone they know received sexual photos or messages on their phones? How did they feel about it and how did they respond?

- **Help** your teens come up with ways to resist pressure to say or do things that make them uncomfortable, even online. Introduce them to www.thatsnotcool.com, a practical, teen-friendly web site that helps young people deal with real life digital issues.

- **Remind** them that once they hit the "send" button, the message or photo is out of their control. At the click of a button that message or photo can be forwarded on… and on… and on… Even a mobile app like Snapchat, which allows the sender to select how long a photo and text can be viewed (between one and ten seconds), provides only the illusion of being fully in control of content once it has been sent.

- **Encourage** your teens to count to 10 before they hit send… and to not send or post any message or photo they're unwilling to have everyone see, including other friends, strangers, the school principal, a younger sibling, a future employer or you.

- **Help** them realize that impulsive decisions can come back to haunt them… and that once they post, send or even forward something, there's no calling it back.

- **Be honest** about possible short- and long-term risks and consequences of sharing inappropriate content, both personal and legal.

- **Help** your teens think about what they can do if someone is sending them sexually explicit messages or photos.

- **Talk** about your expectations for cell phone and web site use. Set appropriate limits.

- **Ask** your teens to consider the impression they make by what they send, post or forward. How do they want others to see them?

- **Talk and listen...** more than once.

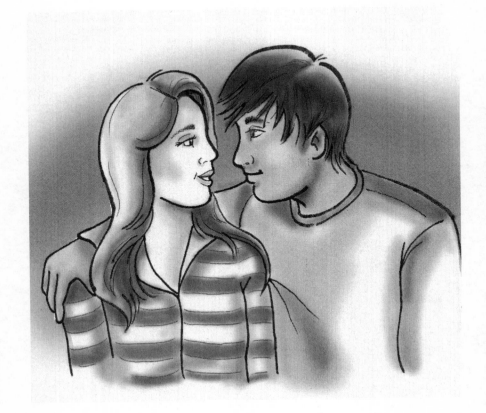

Why should the school take a parent's place as sex educator?

It shouldn't. In an ideal world, parents and kids would talk together about sexual issues with ease, grace and comfort. Conversations would be open; accurate information and values would be shared; healthy attitudes about sexuality would be modeled and encouraged. In an ideal world.

In the real world, both parents and youth want some help with sex education. Most parents recognize it's important that children learn information and skills to understand and appreciate sexuality. During the teenage years, specific sexual health issues become even more pertinent: peer pressure, dating, sexual decision-making, unintended pregnancy, sexually transmitted diseases, HIV and AIDS...

When our kids were younger, "just say no" may have seemed like enough. It's certainly easier when they're 10. You simply say, *"You're not ready for sex."* Period. But what do you say when they're 17 or 18? Most parents realize that "just say no" is an incomplete and insufficient way to address the complexity of sexual issues with teens. Parents are looking to schools, to their faith communities, and to other community resources to work *with* them to educate their children.

State and national polls consistently show that the majority of parents are in favor of having comprehensive sex education taught in schools. If you count yourself among them, think about how you can support your local school in providing effective programs for youth. If your family belongs to a faith community, talk with your pastor, rabbi or other faith leader about how sex education can be provided to young people within that setting. The more we can partner with religious institutions, schools and other trusted community resources in educating young people about healthy sexuality, the better our children will fare.

It's not about anyone *replacing* parents in this important role. It's about *enhancing* the good stuff that happens when caring adults work together to support the health and well-being of youth.

Share your wisdom

Adolescence is not a disease. It is an exciting time of explosive development on many levels. Teens are like chameleons: one day wise, mature and responsible; the next day inappropriate in their behavior and lacking in good judgment. Love and patience are tested to the limits.

It's not a particularly good time for sex to enter the picture. Yet at this stage it often does. Research shows that about 47% of high school students have had sexual intercourse (Youth Risk Behavior Survey, Centers for Disease Control and Prevention, 2013). They are typical, everyday kids from all social, economic and religious backgrounds. Just like the kids next door. Just like *your* kids.

Maybe you should talk... again.

Young people wonder:

What's wrong with teens having sex as long as they're responsible?
What does that mean, "being responsible?" Do you and your children agree on what being responsible looks like... and what it means to be responsible with regard to having sex? Does responsibility go beyond consent and using sexual protection and contraception? Many believe sex is for marriage, or at least for the adult years. Have you shared your beliefs about this with your children? Have you asked them what their thoughts are about this? Whether or not your children hold your same perspective, it's important for them to know how you feel. Urge them to take time to think through what they value.

Ask your teens how they think sex might affect a relationship in both positive and negative ways. How prepared – emotionally and otherwise – do they think young people are to take that on?

If people begin having sex when they're young, they often wind up having more partners over a lifetime. That means a greater chance of being exposed to sexually transmitted diseases (STDs). Condoms and dental dams certainly offer good protection from many STDs, but there is still some level of risk.

Chances are good that you and your teens can talk about many reasons why even responsible teens benefit from delaying sex until they're older.

How can you tell if you're really in love? We know there's a difference between love and sex, right? And we know that sexual attraction creates powerful feelings that are sometimes mistaken for love. The passion of the moment can be astounding. It's easy to get swept away.

Love takes time and effort. People who are in love respect each other, share the most intimate parts of their lives, and communicate about the things that are important to them. Love is supportive and honors agreements; it respects boundaries and doesn't pressure or coerce. *Love may or may not include sex.*

Teens get confused. They live with a language that calls having sex "making love," regardless of the relationship. They presume being "turned on" is the same as being "in love" and is therefore a good reason for "making love." No one has offered to explain the difference.

Talk about the difference with your teens. They may say, *"Really? I already know this stuff!"* Be persistent. Say something like, *"I know you do, but bear with me, OK? I'm checking in to be sure I've got it straight."*

At some point your teens will be making choices about sex. Regardless of when that happens, they need to understand the difference between things like love, infatuation and attraction, and how those feelings influence their sexual decision-making.

In search of understanding

When Alec's son Jack told his dad he needed to talk with him about a friend he was worried about, Alec got a little nervous. As a kid, whenever Alec was troubled and needed answers, he never admitted he was the one with the issue. It was always, *"I've got this 'friend,' and he's got this problem..."* So going into the conversation with Jack, Alec felt just a bit concerned.

"He's gay, Dad," Jack stated, *"and he doesn't want to tell his family."*

"Who is it?" Alec asked, almost too quickly. What he wanted to say was: *"Jack, who are we really talking about here?"* But Alec contained himself. He appreciated that Jack felt he could talk to him, no matter what. Alec didn't want to say or do anything that might shut down this conversation.

Jack replied, *"I don't want to say, Dad. I just need to talk about it. There's a lot of gay bashing that goes on at school. Sometimes it's more like off-handed comments and jokes. Maybe people just don't get what it's all about. I'm not sure I understand it."*

Alec told Jack all he knew about the subject, which he confessed wasn't much. He told Jack that many children and teens have some kind of sexual experience with people of the same gender – including "playing doctor" when they're younger and sexual touching, feelings of attraction and sexual fantasies when they get older. Such experiences and feelings are common, normal, and may or may not have anything to do with being gay.

Alec told his son, *"There are a lot of theories, Jack, and there's been a lot of research, but no one knows what 'causes' someone to be either gay or straight. It's likely a complicated combination of lots of different factors. Evidence shows that being gay – or being straight, for that matter – isn't a choice. We may not understand... and we don't have to. Relationships, whether gay, lesbian or heterosexual, can be loving and fulfilling. It's important to respect that."*

Alec emphasized that it's wrong to mistreat or discriminate against people because of their sexual orientation or gender identity. In fact, there are laws that provide some protection. He reminded Jack that sexual orientation isn't contagious. Having a gay or straight teacher, coach, best friend or even a parent doesn't "turn" someone gay or straight.

It turned out Jack really *was* asking about a friend. But what if he wasn't? There are many young people out there feeling confused, ashamed and alienated from their peers. They may be unable to express who they are, fear judgment or rejection from family and friends, and have no one to turn to about their concerns. Lesbian, gay, bisexual and transgender youth often feel unacknowledged at best, and are often discriminated against, harassed, or far worse. Think about it... sex education, if it happens at all, is typically phrased in heterosexual terms. Gender options are either male or female... you check which box you belong in. But what if neither of those boxes fits who you are or how you identify?

Jack and others like him can be supportive by making themselves available to listen and care; speaking up and taking action (within limits of personal safety) in the face of offensive remarks, harassment and bullying; and suggesting helpful resources such as:

- It Gets Better Project – www.itgetsbetter.org

- PFLAG (Parents, Families and Friends of Lesbians and Gays) – www.pflag.org

- Gay, Lesbian & Straight Education Network – www.glsen.org

- Gender Spectrum – www.genderspectrum.org

- Be an Active Bystander and Bystander Intervention Playbook – www.stopabuse.vt.edu

When we avoid honest conversations about sexual orientation or gender identity, we allow for continued misunderstanding, mistrust, fear and isolation. Parents: Jack, his friend and all those like him encourage you to speak with your teens.

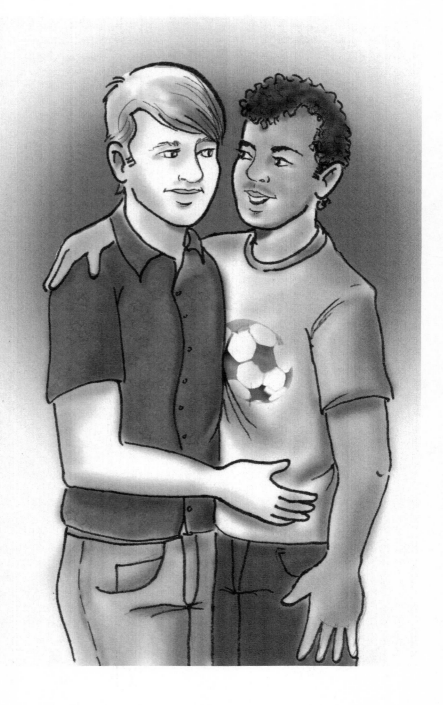

Yet another challenge

What if...

As usual, you checked to make sure there was nothing left in the pockets of your son's pants before tossing them into the wash. You found a condom.

What if...

Rushing off for school, your daughter dropped her purse and the contents scattered across the floor. There was a folded up brochure about teen birth control services provided by the local Planned Parenthood.

How does a parent respond to a suspicion that their 17-year-old might be having sex? What should they do? And *not* do?

First: *breathe*... slowly, deeply... take time to move past the alarm or whatever that initial gut reaction might be. Remind yourself that the conversation you need to have with your teen will be more productive once you've calmed down and thought things through.

Consider the facts: Your son has a condom. Is it for use or show? Carrying a condom might be seen as a mark of sexual experience among his peers. Then again, maybe he is having sex.

And the brochure from Planned Parenthood? It's possible your daughter picked it up in health class the day a guest speaker came in to talk about teen pregnancy. Maybe it's for a school assignment. Then again, maybe she is having sex.

If you find yourself questioning whether your teen is having sex, be honest with them about it. Tell them — with as much calm as you can muster — what you found or saw or heard that left you wondering. Listen to what they have to say. Their response may be *very* brief... like one word. That's OK. Try to listen and not default to a lecture.

Let your teen know that this conversation is about more than whether or not you approve. It's about ensuring that whatever decision they've made about sex, it is in fact *their* decision, and that they are well informed, caring and thoughtful about it. Of course, remind them of your values and what you hope for them with regard to having sex at this age.

If it turns out your suspicion is correct, avoid comments like, *"How could you do this?"* or *"I'm so disappointed in you."* Blaming, shaming or guilt-tripping will not help – in fact, it can bring a pretty quick end to any discussion you hope to have. Focus on the *behavior.* If you think it's inappropriate or unwise or risky for your teen to have sex, say that. And talk about why you believe that.

Ask your teen about the circumstances and the reasons they've made that choice. What is the status of the relationship and the level of commitment? Why has sex become part of the relationship? Is there pressure to have sex? Are they using protection carefully to avoid sexually transmitted diseases, and contraception if needed? *Consistently affirm that you love and support your child even if you disagree with their behavior.*

Resist the urge to forbid your teen to see their partner again. This often just drives the relationship underground. Threats and ultimatums can bring resentment, anger, resistance... none of which serve to keep the dialogue open so you can guide your child in making wise, safe choices.

Though parents may not approve of the behavior, they still have a responsibility to make sure their children are informed and thoughtful with their choice to have a sexual relationship. Understanding possible outcomes and risks, knowing the laws, being aware of sexual and reproductive health services in the community... this information is important to making healthy sexual decisions, just as values and beliefs are.

In the end, your teen may continue to be sexually active. S/he may choose to reconsider. Either way, your connection and guidance, which are so necessary to your child's well-being, can continue only if you keep those lines of communication open.

What to do?!

Young people may think that the only choice to be made about sex is, *"Should I or shouldn't I?"* Sexual decision-making involves a lot more than merely deciding whether to have sex, and if so, when and with whom. Life after high school brings increasing opportunities to engage in sexual behavior. For some, it can be incredibly complicated... so many conflicting messages, from "just say no" to "just do it!" No wonder it's confusing.

Can you say to your teen:

— *"Your body belongs to you. You decide how to express yourself, sexually and otherwise. Right now, you have the ability to say yes or no to a range of sexual behaviors. You may feel a strong influence from your peers, your parents or your faith to make a particular decision. Bottom line is, it's up to you. Whatever you decide, choose thoughtfully."*

— *"Consider how you make your decisions. If it's by impulse, how's that going to work out for you? If your judgment is clouded (by drugs, alcohol, stress, etc.), how might that affect your decisions?"*

— *"If you let someone else decide for you, do you risk going against what you really want or believe? If you don't clearly make and express a decision, could this give someone else the chance to step in and decide for you?"*

— *"If you evaluate options and then decide, how might that increase your power to make choices that are consistent with your personal values?"*

Important decisions in life deserve careful consideration. Help your teen appreciate that empowerment, freedom and self-respect come from taking charge of one's life choices.

A letter of love

Cass and Dale's son Kevin is a high school senior. What a landmark. They recognize that this is Kevin's final year home with them – he's off to college in a few months. As they prepare to launch this young man into the world on his own, they remember all the talks they had... or didn't have... or wish they'd had with Kevin about sex. They want to keep the conversation open as he moves into the next chapter of his life.

Sexuality is such a complex issue at any age. Cass and Dale understand that some of the greatest challenges lie ahead – on the college campus and beyond. They want Kevin to be prepared. So they wrote him a letter (really old school, right?) and tucked it away in one of the duffel bags Kevin is packing off to school at the end of summer. He'll probably roll his eyes when he finds it, which is fine with them as long as he also takes the message to heart.

It takes extra effort to talk with a 12th-grader about sex. There are so many shades of gray, "what ifs" and differing opinions. Emotions run high; discomfort sets in quickly. Sometimes it's easier to just forget it, cross your fingers and hope you've already covered it all. But Kevin's parents didn't want to do that. They wanted to take one more opportunity through this letter:

Dear Kevin,

You're growing into a handsome, bright and sexy young man. Watching you fills us with love and pride – plus, we confess, a bit of worry. But then, do parents *ever* stop worrying about their kids?

It's difficult to accept you as the sexy young man that you are – and frankly, hard to ignore. As you go through the process of understanding yourself as a sexual person, please think about the beliefs and values we have shared with you over the years. We hope you take the time you need to make wise choices that are right for you. Your decisions about sex are yours and yours alone. Whatever you choose, choose responsibly.

We expect you to be thoughtful, respectful and honorable in your sexual decision-making, Kevin. Love and sex are not one and the same... don't confuse them or misrepresent them to another.

We expect that you will make sexual decisions that are positive and affirming... not ones that exploit either yourself or others. We respect that some of your beliefs may differ from ours. We trust that you have taken the time to carefully sort out what you value and hold to be true. We also trust that you will act on your values... for only then will you feel self-respect.

We hope you feel that you can come to us if you find yourself confused, hurt or stuck on any issue you're struggling to resolve, whether it's related to sex, relationships, school... whatever.

Remember we love you very much, Kevin, and are proud to be your parents.

Communication review: twenty pocket tips for parents

In no particular order (except maybe the first one):

- Start early – but if you haven't, start now.

- Seize the teachable moments.

- Sound bites work better than sermons.

- Talk about sexuality, not just sex.

- Be willing to initiate conversations.

- Listen.

- Anticipate and plan ahead.

- Be inclusive and open to the possibility that your child has another sense about their sexual orientation and/or gender identity than you do.

- Share information about the pleasures, joys and intimacy of sex – not just the risks and dangers.

- Have conversations about when saying yes makes sense.

- Hear what your children have to say – what they think and value.

- Make it safe for your children to talk with you.

- Share facts about sexual issues along with your beliefs and values.

- Set an example through your actions, not just with your words.

- Trust that your children are capable of making choices that are good for them.

- Trust that your children really do want to hear what you have to say about these issues.

- Remind your children frequently that you love them, no matter what.

- Respond with delight. Be mindful of your words, tone and body language.

- Be realistic, be accepting and don't beat yourself up.

- Raise your children to be good friends and caring partners.

Resource Section

Web sites for parents

- **Families Are Talking/La familia habla –**
www.familiesaretalking.org – This newsletter series from the Sex Information and Education Council of the U.S. (SIECUS) offers support to parents and caregivers on talking with children about sexual issues.

- **Parents Sex Ed Center –**
www.advocatesforyouth.org/parents – This is part of the Advocates for Youth web site and provides information for talking with children about sexual issues.

- **Talking with Kids about Tough Issues –**
www.talkingwithkids.org – Helpful tips and strategies from Children Now support parents and caregivers in talking with young people ages 8 to 12 about a number of tough issues, including sexuality and relationships.

- **Let's Talk** –
www.plannedparenthood.org/parents – Planned Parenthood Federation of America's web site provides tools for parents that help with setting boundaries, talking with kids about sex and sexuality, parenting LGBT and questioning kids, and much more.

- **PFLAG (Parents, Families and Friends of Lesbians and Gays)** –
www.pflag.org – This national family and ally organization has chapters throughout the country, providing support, education and advocacy. Search for local PFLAG chapters from this site.

- **Accord Alliance** –
www.accordalliance.org – This web site includes a detailed Handbook for Parents designed for parents and others who have children with disorders of sex development (DSD). The handbook provides information and ideas for helping children with DSD to adapt and thrive in their lives.

- **National Campaign to Prevent Teen and Unplanned Pregnancy** –
www.thenationalcampaign.org – This web site includes access to a significant number of online resources including research reports, publications, fact sheets, podcasts and more.

- **Safe Teens** –
www.safeteens.com – While designed for teens, this site also includes a "Parents' Corner" that offers helpful strategies for talking with teens.

Web sites for young people

- **www.plannedparenthood.org/info-for-teens** –
Provides accurate information for teens on many different areas of healthy sexuality in a fun and friendly format.

- **www.youthresource.com** –
A web site by and for lesbian, gay, bisexual, transgender and questioning youth.

- **www.loveisrespect.org** –
This web site fosters healthy dating attitudes and relationships and creates a safe space for young people to access information and help.

- **www.amplifyyourvoice.org** –
Amplify is a youth activism project of Advocates for Youth. Advocates for Youth champions efforts to help young people make informed and responsible decisions about their reproductive and sexual health.

- **www.sexetc.org** –
A web site and free newsletter produced for teens by teens. Writers take on all different angles of preventing pregnancy and disease transmission.

- **www.iwannaknow.org** –
Sponsored by the American Sexual Health Association, this site offers information on various topics having to do with healthy sexuality.

- **www.thatsnotcool.com** –
This web site raises awareness for youth about healthy friendships/relationships and what you can do if you (or your friend) are in an unhealthy one.

Books

- **What Makes a Baby**
Cory Silverberg
Seven Stories Press

- **Bellybuttons Are Navels**
Mark Schoen
BookSurge

- **Beyond the Big Talk: Every Parent's Guide to Raising Sexually Healthy Teens – From Middle School to High School and Beyond**
Debra Haffner
Newmarket Press

- **Caution: Do Not Open Until Puberty! An Introduction to Sexuality for Young Adults with Disabilities**
Rick Enrigh
Thames Valley Children's Centre

- **Happy Birth Day!**
Robie H. Harris
Candlewick Press

- **It's Perfectly Normal: Changing Bodies, Growing Up, Sex, and Sexual Health**
Robie H. Harris
Candlewick Press

- **It's So Amazing! A Book about Eggs, Sperm, Birth, Babies, and Families**
Robie H. Harris
Candlewick Press

- **My Body, My Self for Boys: The "What's Happening to My Body?" Workbook for Boys**
Lynda Madaras & Area Madaras
Newmarket Press

- **My Body, My Self For Girls: The "What's Happening to My Body?" Workbook**
Lynda Madaras & Area Madaras
Newmarket Press

- **The What's Happening to My Body? Book for Boys: A Growing Up Guide for Parents and Sons**
Lynda Madaras & Dane Saavedra
Newmarket Press

- **"What's Happening to My Body?" Book for Girls: A Growing-Up Guide for Parents and Daughters**
Lynda Madaras & Area Madaras
Newmarket Press

- **Words Can Work: When Talking with Kids about Sexual Health**
Jeanne Blake
Family Health Productions, Inc.

Index

Made in the USA
Lexington, KY
19 June 2017